Acupuncture for Longevity

Li Zheng and Changhong Zhou PhD.

Edited by Steven Zhou

Also by Li Zheng and Changhong Zhou

Acupuncture and Hormone Balance

Acupuncture and Infertility

Erectile Dysfunction and Prostate Problems

Acupuncture and Eye Health

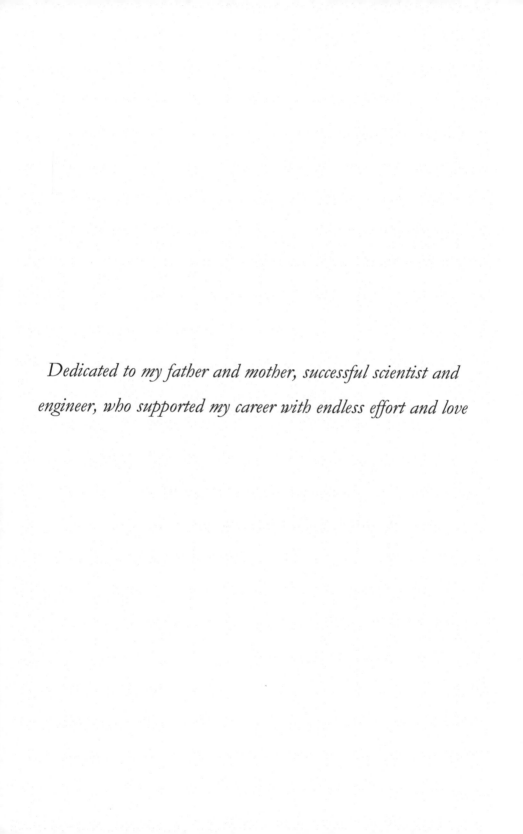

Dedicated to my father and mother, successful scientist and engineer, who supported my career with endless effort and love

Acknowledgements

I would like to thank my father, Zheng, ZhiZhen, for his encouragement, endless love and help. He was dedicated to his family and his work never thinking of his own needs. He grew up in a big family and was one of the smartest and healthiest children. Since his childhood, he had been taking care of his parents and siblings. By his own effort, he entered the most prestigious Beijing University. From that time on, his life's work became research into more reliable predictions of earthquakes and tornados.

Even though he wrote five books, more than 100 papers, and mentored more than 10 graduate students, he never stopped working. His only satisfaction was to make contributions to his profession and his family. He helped me choose the right career and encouraged me to come to America. During my residence in Dong Zhi Men Hospital, the affiliated hospital of the Beijing University of Chinese Medicine, he took care of my daughter Iris and my son Steven. Now Iris is a mature, responsible, lawyer, who graduated from Harvard Law School. Even during his chemotherapy, he made his effort to teach Steven math. Steven represented Wellesley Middle School on the state math competition for the first time in 2012. During my Ph. D study, my father came to America to help me take care of my very sick son Steven and cook three meals a day for my family. I still remember the way he held Steven with both his arms for hours in order to let Steven get some sleep when he was covered with rashes and his body was swelling from his sickness. Later he took this sick child with a heart problem to China and brought him back healthy two years later.

When I first set up my own clinic, my dad used his own hands to fix the furniture and electronics. He never asked for one single cent from me. He had been a strong believer in acupuncture and Chinese herbal medicine. He devoted his last nine years of his life to alternative medicine hoping to use his effort to relieve other people's suffering, but he forgot to take care of himself. I was too busy to persuade him to get regular X-rays when he had repetitive coughing every winter. In order to save my time, he had tried not to bother me until he found out he had difficulty breathing. After he was diagnosed as stage IV lung cancer, he never complained.

He religiously took herbs and had acupuncture treatments every day until the last few days he lived in this world. When he had severe headaches and ear ringing, he refused to use morphine; instead it was acupuncture that helped him to feel more comfortable until the last two days before he passed away. From my father's life experiences, I learned how to become a successful person using my own effort. On the other hand, I learned that we have to reach a balance between taking care of other people and ourselves. If you only think about yourself, you can not achieve anything in your life; if you make every effort to make other people healthy and happy, by the end, you may endanger your own health and your suffering will make your family members sad. Not only will you not enjoy your life, but you may not be able to help other people in the long run.

My dad was diagnosed with late stage lung cancer after he came back from taking care of my brother. The oncologist only gave him three months to live. My dad did not blame anybody; instead he took herbs and acupuncture every day. It is amazing that he never developed neuropathy or lung infection during his chemotherapy. His tumor was shrinking for a while combining acupuncture, herbs and chemotherapy. He used his courage and persistency to create a miracle in lung cancer treatment history: his oxygen saturation was normal even after the majority of his lungs were eaten up by the cancer cells. He unfortunately did not pay attention to his diet, and due to many years of deficiency of vitamins and minerals, he developed anxiety, which caused his immune function to be out of balance. He could have lived to his eighties or nineties, but he used all of his energy to serve his profession and other people. Eventually his body functions were worn down.

My dad had been such a motivated person that whenever he started a project, he wanted to finish it as soon as possible, and then he would start the next one. He lived at such a fast pace that his body could not catch up with his thoughts after he passed age 65. He did not sleep well for his last ten years, and his immune function lost control over the cancer cells. In his last few months in this world, he told me to slow down, be generous with people and be happy. He taught me not expect patients to change quickly even though my suggestions would benefit their health. He wanted me to be more patient. He taught me to focus on whatever I am doing and not get distracted by talking too much.

I thank my dad for his strong beliefs in Chinese medicine. I thank him because he set a good example by working hard and never expected a reward, except the joy of work itself. As I observed his life I learned lessons not specifically intended: if we do not take care of ourselves, nobody else can, that if we want to be happy and healthy, we have to slow down to enjoy everything we do and we must appreciate our friends, our family, and the people who come into our lives for only an instant.

Foreword

Dr. Li Zheng has accumulated considerable perspective about personal health care through her studies of traditional Chinese medicine, her PhD coursework and research, and her clinical experience over many years as a health care advisor and provider. In this book, she shares her insights about numerous aspects of human health and offers many practical suggestions for how to achieve and maintain good health. Background discussion is presented about a variety of prevalent health concerns, and interesting case studies, drawn from Dr. Zheng's extensive clinical experiences, provide examples of how to overcome specific health problems, by lifestyle changes, acupuncture, and/or herbal remedies.

Donald A. Godfrey

Department of Neurology and Division of Otolaryngology & Dentistry, Department of Surgery

Mail Stop 1195

University of Toledo College of Medicine

3000 Arlington Avenue

Toledo, Ohio 43614

Table of Contents

Introduction

Every organ and system of the body has one stimulating (Yang) and one relaxing (Yin) component that complement and balance each other. For instance, our nervous system consists of the "fight or flight" sympathetic nervous systems (SNS) – the Yang side, which handles daily stress, and of the relaxing Yin part called the parasympathetic nervous system (PNS), which controls digestion and repair. These two halves become dominant during different times of the day and in different seasons, at each moment trying to attain a harmonious balance. If we lose balance for too long, certain organ functions, whether digestive, immune, or nervous, will be damaged.

Each individual has a different constitution because they each inherited a different genome. People with Yin-type constitution display slow or moderate metabolism and a more laid back personality. Usually, they have a relatively stronger PNS, so they can relax easily without over-thinking. Furthermore, they sleep very well – even with coffee - and absorb food more efficiently because they have little trouble blocking out troubling thoughts. On the other hand, they tend to gain weight and especially if they sit on the couch watching TV and snacking, they are the best candidates for obesity. From a survival point of view, this type of constitution saves a lot of energy by sleeping well and thinking less, but if they do eat the wrong foods and become obese, they have great difficulty loosing weight. Although certain amounts of fat help us cope with environmental stresses such as hunger, cold, and infection, if too much is present, these benefits will be compromised by the overburdening of the heart and joints and the excess of estrogen and different toxins stored in fat tissues.

People with Yang-type constitution have higher metabolic rates and stronger SNS, tend to over-think, and are very sensitive to environmental changes. Therefore, Yang-type individuals frequently develop panic attacks under stress, because once their "fight or flight system" is triggered, it tends to go on and on until balance between the Yin and the Yang sides of the nervous system is somehow restored. Yang-type people usually sleep very little or not very deeply because they are always active mentally or physically, unable to sit down and relax. Their muscles tend to be tight, and although they have strong appetites, their constant movements burn most of their calories. Furthermore, because their SNS is dominant, their intestines absorb nutrients less efficiently than those of Yin-type people. Yang-type bodies tend to develop insomnia, heart problems, high blood pressure, adrenal fatigue, panic attacks, cancer, and autoimmune diseases if they do not train their bodies to slow down and get enough rest.

Then, does this mean that every Yin-type or every Yang-type body will show the same symptoms? The answer is no. For example, while some Yang-type people have more allergies, others develop facial flushing and still others tend to have very cold hands and feet and easily disturbed sleep. However, they do all share one characteristic: a tendency to overreact to stress and environmental changes. If you realize that you have this constitution, you will need to choose the right exercises, eat the right food, and drink the right beverages, which means staying away from too much coffee, too much alcohol, and too much spicy food. You will have to try hard to maintain the balance of your nervous system. For instance, if two cups of coffee make your jittery, try one cup instead or substitute it with green tea. If arguing with people causes you to sweat, try avoiding it. If you really love red wine, drink it only on weekends, which would not only make this event seem more special but would also prevent the alcohol from constantly interrupting the balance of your nervous system to the point that your body can no longer compensate.

On the other hand, a Yin-type constitution handles stress better because his or her metabolism is slower. In America, however, Yin-types can become easily addicted to sugar, coffee, alcohol, and tobacco as they have the freedom to eat whenever and whatever they want until systematic inflammation causes diabetes, neuropathy, colon cancer, and other detrimental diseases. Because Yin-type bodies respond to harmful materials more slowly, oftentimes they do not notice the damage until it is too late.

Balance is the key to achieving longevity and success. In this book, I will introduce self-healing methods for some of the most commonly seen diseases in our modern society and explore the factors that cause such imbalances. For the practitioner's convenience, I will also list effective Chinese herbal formulae and acupuncture points that, in my clinical experience, achieve the best therapeutic effect.

Chapter One

Allergies

I take this problem very personally. I, Li Zheng, suffer from allergies. Too much stress and my immune function goes crazy! Wine or beer triggers my allergies. Acid reflux, a constricted throat, and rashes afflict me. I understand, very personally, the impact of allergies. Sometimes they can be merely annoying, like the constant dripping of a runny nose, but often the problem can dramatically affect the quality of your life. I'm going to tell you about a patient of mine who had such a problem. Luckily it was not a life or death situation for him, but for many this problem . . . is . . . a . . .KILLER.

My patient was a public person so I'm going to change his name for privacy reasons; let's call him Benny Rosa. At the time, he was a 45-year-old successful businessman and a former professional athlete. He is still popular enough that you might even know him by reputation. Let's just say he is a sports figure in the Boston area. He was referred to me by a mutual friend from the medical field.

He had been very conscious about his health and had been a vegetarian since college. Therefore, nuts had become one of his main sources of protein. He had such strong personal discipline that he never ate any junk food and seldom over-ate. His weight had remained stable from his twenties to his forties. He came to see me in 2003 for the simple reason that he wanted to stay healthy as he grew older. He took acupuncture treatments once a month to fine-tune his bodily functions and to make him more energetic and efficient. I found that if I did electro-acupuncture late in the evening, he would not be able to get a sound sleep that night. He would still be very energetic, however, the next day because of the temporary increase in secretion of cortisol from his adrenal gland. The only issue he had was the wart on the bottom of his left foot, which he had been trying to get rid of in many ways. The wart was caused by a viral infection. I used certain acupuncture points to strengthen his immune function to fight the viral infection, and then applied indirect moxa (burning one kind of herb called mugwort) above his foot area. After 6 treatments, his wart was completely gone. He then ceased treatments for one year because of some family issues.

Then something strange happened: he developed hives. No one knew why. I told him to reduce his intake of nuts, especially peanuts. He said that his favorites were almonds. However, he continued eating almonds, and the rashes came and went while he was taking anti-histamine medication. Why didn't he listen to me? Most of his rashes were distributed on his back. They started at night and quickly disappeared during the day. Gradually, the rashes appeared more frequently and sometimes even showed up on his lips or around his eyes. This development made him very uncomfortable and sometimes embarrassed because he had to deal with clients, vendors, and peers all day long. Around this time he also complained of digestion problems.

It is unusual for me to be treating someone who eats well but has diet-related health problems. This case interested me because of this fact. Was the problem possibly related to food allergies? Why hadn't he had this problem before? What had changed? I had so many questions, yet so few answers at this point.

My Diagnosis: What did I tell Benny Rosa?

Initially, when he took anti-histamine, the rashes would disappear within a couple of hours. As time went on, however, it would take a whole day for the rashes to diminish. After this, the condition lasted for a couple of months, and he finally decided to try acupuncture. I also prescribed certain herbs to help his digestion and to clear his body of toxins, because he always had a thick coating on his tongue and bad breath, which indicated that his digestion needed to be optimized. I always look for the simplest solution that will cause the fewest side effects yet fix the problem. Often it is a hybrid of efforts but always based on scientific proof and clinical experiences.

This indigestion may have been associated with nuts, because nut protein is very hard to digest. While we were adjusting his herbal formula, he had 5 acupuncture treatments within 3 weeks, targeting this issue.

What happened to Benny Rosa?

I began to feel that the treatment was working. It is a little difficult for a client to get better if he or she doesn't follow my advice. He was starting to listen to me.

In the meantime, he stopped eating nuts of all kinds, including peanuts for a few weeks. Interestingly, I also discovered in conversation that his wife used peanut oil to cook. I talk and talk so much to my patients that I often find out these hidden facts that, left undiscovered, would prolong the medical problem, or prevent me from ever getting to the root cause. I say to myself AHA, THE MISSING CLUE. So I asked him to stop using peanut oil. He took herbs for a week and gradually stopped the anti-histamine medication. Slowly he started to see improvement. He was amazed. He said, "Li, if I had known before that this could be fixed this fast, I would have listened to every instruction you gave me. I am now a true believer". I guess it takes a while to change people's habits, but some improvement in symptoms helps to speed up the changes. His hives were completely gone within two weeks of treatments. After 5 weeks, he began re-introducing almonds

4

little by little, and so far his hives have not returned. His digestion problems disappeared as well. I guess the success a person like Benny achieved in his life resulted from a large amount of ego and self-reliance. In his case, he would have gotten healthier faster had he had a little less self-reliance and a little more reliance on scientific evidence.

What causes peanut allergies?

Generally speaking, peanut protein is much harder to digest in the stomach than other proteins. If a person has healthy digestion and eats nuts infrequently, they can be broken down to small amino acids and absorbed as a valuable nutrient. If a person eats a large quantity of nuts or drinks too much soda, or if his stress level is too high, the protein is only partially digested, and the bigger molecules can stimulate the body to produce antibodies, which can trigger severe allergies. In Chinese medical theory, it is thought that antibiotics impair digestive function, so long-term usage of antibiotics can lead to indigestion of protein. Again, digestion plays a critical role in the development of food allergies. New research shows that when scientists disable one of the genes in peanuts, people do not develop severe allergies. This indicates that certain genetic components in peanuts are key factors in the development of human allergies.

In the case of Benny Rosa, who had not been previously allergic to nuts, why did he suddenly develop hives, even though he maintained a very healthy lifestyle? Perhaps it was associated with age-related changes in digestion. When we pass a certain age, our enzymes do not function as well as before. If he ate the same amount of nuts as he did in his younger years, his digestive system may not be able to process all this food as well. The undigested nut protein can lead to allergies. Another possibility is that his stress level may have been high at that time, so that his hormones got out of balance. His cortisol level may have dropped after coping with stress for a long time, which also could have compromised his body's anti-allergy function. He later told me that his sleep patterns had changed recently. He used to be able to sleep for 8 hours straight without getting up to go to the bathroom. However, for the past couple of months, he woke up once or twice each night to use the bathroom. Sometimes, he could not go back to sleep afterwards. This sleep problem also indicates that his hormones had started changing because his cortisol, serotonin or melatonin wasn't at its optimal level.

In Chinese medicine, we have a theory saying that our bodies go through major changes every 5 years after we reach 50 years of age. We have to adjust our lifestyles accordingly. For example, a CEO of a biotech company drank coffee for more than 20 years without experiencing any problems. When he turned 40, he started vomiting every time he drank coffee. If he wanted to continue being an active CEO, he had to stop drinking coffee. Now, he only consumes green tea in moderation as his stimulant.

Modern medicine can save people's lives from severe allergic reactions such as anaphylactic shock. When allergists treat food allergies, they first prescribe anti-histamine medication, then cortisol. If these don't work, they will give allergy shots and suggest that the patient avoid all foods to which he or she may possibly be allergic. In most cases, following this protocol, children's allergies become worse and worse if they do not have a healthy lifestyle. Eventually, they may have to carry an EpiPen everywhere to protect them from dying of an anaphylactic shock.

My strategy is to find the root cause of an allergy and then use appropriate preventative methods and changes of lifestyle. If you cannot get rid of your allergies in this way, try Chinese herbal medicines to clear up chronic inflammation and to restore balance of your immune system. After your symptoms completely disappear, gradually re-introduce the food you are allergic to in very small amounts once or twice a week. For some children for whom even the smell of peanuts or the accidental consumption of foods containing a trivial amount of peanut oil can lead to anaphylactic shock, if they follow the above advice, I am fairly sure that they will grow out of this dangerous condition, even though they may never be able to eat real peanuts.

I was never allergic to peanuts before I came to America. During my third year in the U.S., I developed a choking sensation, hives and runny nose if I ate too many nuts. I had no problem breathing or swallowing but felt as if something was stuck in my throat, and the constant contraction of my esophagus drove me crazy at night. I took Chinese herbs for 8 months the last time I had an allergic episode with peanuts and red wine. I also could not eat seafood, nuts or spicy food while I had my allergies. My allergies went away 8 years ago, and now I can eat small amounts of various nuts once or twice a week. I still don't dare to try red wine, however.

How to Prevent Allergies?

1. Drink enough water to prevent dehydration and to help your body discharge environmental toxins. Chemical toxins can sensitize your body. Dehydration can lead to histamine release, which is one of the reasons why athletes may have asthma attacks during or after training or races.

2. Avoid seafood or nuts during periods of allergic reactions. Reintroduce them little by little after the allergies are gone. When you have a weak digestive system, try to eat easily digested food because your stomach may not be able to digest seafood or nut protein thoroughly if it is not functioning well. The undigested protein can trigger the allergic reaction.

3. Check your medications, because some medications may aggravate allergies. Non-steroid, anti-inflammatory medications and antibiotics are the drugs most commonly associated with hives. Selective

serotonin re-uptake inhibitors (SSRI), angiotensin-converting enzyme inhibitors (ACEI), and systemic anti-fungal medications have also been reported to cause rashes. One woman told me that after she received chemotherapy treatment for breast cancer, she developed chronic hives, lasting more than a year. One day, she suffered from a headache, took one tablet of aspirin, and was then rushed to the emergency room because her throat almost closed up. Later, an allergist told her that she should not take aspirin if she has hives.

4. Avoid long-term use of antibiotics; try other ways to treat acne. For example, my daughter's friends told me that when they cut down on sweets, ate less greasy, spicy food, and drank more water, their acne became much better. Teenager acne is due to hormone fluctuation. If they eat enough vegetables, drink more water, and avoid simple sugars, their bodies are better able to discharge extra hormone metabolites.

5. If you have never eaten a certain kind of food before, especially during childhood, try to introduce it little by little. Do not eat it every day; start by testing it out no more than twice a week. If you find that you have itchy sensations, rashes, or acid reflux, stop eating it for a while and see if the symptoms clear up.

6. Do not over-eat any kind of food, such as strawberries or nuts. You should have as many choices as possible, with moderate

amounts of each kind. The theory here is that small amounts of food will desensitize the body whereas large amounts could do the opposite. Allergy shots operate by the same mechanism. Some allergists treat allergies by introducing sublingual drops that contain many kinds of allergens in small amounts.

7. Try to protect children less than 2 years of age from bacterial or viral infections because their immune functions are not yet fully developed. If they do get an infection, do not use antibiotics for too long. Certain herbs have very good anti-bacterial and anti-viral effects, as proven by both human experience and scientific research.

8. Feed children home-made foods as much as you can, especially when they are sick and have weak digestive functions. Try to avoid feeding kids barbecued meat; well-cooked meat has a much smaller chance of inducing food allergies. Parents should start baby food as early as 6 months of age to raise a healthy child.

9. Get plenty of sleep. Remember that histamine release is closely related with the sleep-wake cycle. I have found that children who are always alert and have too much energy tend to develop various kinds of allergies due to the high levels of histamine circulating in their bodies.

10. Avoid intense exercises (such as running) if you have an allergic condition, because it can stimulate the release of adrenaline and

temporarily lower the cortisol level, thus aggravating the itchy sensation. Try more relaxing exercises such as Tai Ji and Qi Gong to lower histamine release.

11. Reduce your stress level as much as possible. Every kind of disease can be aggravated by stress. I.J. Elenkov et al. at the National Institutes of Health in Bethesda, Maryland, localized a corticotropin-releasing hormone (CRH) in a part of the brain called the hypothalamus. This hormone stimulates the adrenal glands to produce more cortisol to fight stress. In humans, CRH is found in the inflamed tissues of patients with severe autoimmune diseases. These researchers demonstrated that CRH activates mast cells, leading to the release of histamine, which ends in fluid leaking from blood vessels. Thus, the activation of the stress system through the direct and indirect effects of CRH may influence the susceptibility of an individual to certain autoimmune diseases, allergies, infection, or even cancer.

12. If you currently have allergies, do not drink red wine or any kind of alcohol, which can stimulate the body to produce more histamine. You can resume drinking once your allergic symptoms are gone.

13. Maintain regular bowel movements. Constipation can make allergies worse because toxic materials stay in the intestines for days and may be reabsorbed into the blood stream.

11

14. Try to avoid extreme hunger, as this may aggravate allergic symptoms. Clinically, when people have rashes, extreme hunger makes them feel itchy everywhere. P. Clementsen of the University of Copenhagen, Denmark, studied histamine release in white blood cell suspensions from normal individuals and from patients allergic to house dust mites or birch pollen. He found that the influenza A virus enhances histamine release from one kind of white blood cell, the basophil, but that sugars can abolish this effect by blocking the binding site on the cell membrane. If your blood sugar level drops too low, it may facilitate histamine release enhanced by other factors such as a viral infection.

15. Avoid a high salt diet, which can lead to dehydration and histamine release. When your body tries to discharge extra salt, the salt draws out huge amounts of water from your body. That is why the more soda you drink, the thirstier you are.

16. Improve your digestion by adding turnip or daikon into your soup. You can also soak tangerine peels in hot water for 5 to 10 minutes, and then drink the water. For tea drinkers, you can choose barley green tea.

17. Add apple cider vinegar to your salad or simply add one tea spoon of it to 5 ounces water and drink it twice to three times a day, depending on how determined you are to get better. You will need to rinse your mouth with water after drinking the vinegar.

Bring This to Your Traditional Chinese Medicine Doctor

Chinese Herbal Formula:

Sheng Di 10g, Mu Dan Pi 10g, Xuan Shen 15g, Mai Dong 10g, Jin Yin Hua 6g, Lian Qiao 6g, Ban Xia 10g, Chi Shao 15g, Zhi Gan Cao 6g, Chan Yi 6g, Fu Ping 10g, Fu Ling 12g.

The patient should take this formula first thing in the morning; within half an hour, your itchy sensation will be gone. You will not scratch the itchy area during the day, which will speed up the clearing of hives. The second dose should be half an hour before your dinner time. When you do not feel itchy after the second dose, you can have longer deep sleep, which drastically lowers your histamine level and boosts your cortisol level. Your body can fight the allergies or inflammation more efficiently during the daytime.

Acupuncture points:

ST43: On the dorsum of the foot, in the depression distal to the junction of the second and third metatarsal bones.

UB12: 1.5 cun lateral to the lower border of the spinous process of the 2nd thoracic vertebra.

UB13: 1.5 cun lateral to the lower border of the spinous process of the 3rd thoracic vertebra.

UB44: 3 cun lateral to the lower border of the spinous process of the 5th thoracic vertebra.

CV14: On the anterior median line of the upper abdomen, 6.0 cun above the bellybutton.

Bai Chong Wo: 3 cun superior to the medial end of the patella

Chapter Two

Acid Reflux

W hat is acid reflux? I bet you've seen a few commercials on TV that sells drugs to help. You may have, on occasion, tasted something acidic in your throat. Some people have that taste *all the time*. Those drugs you see advertised might work . . . with side effects that they mention at the end, very fast.

Chinese medicine looks at the underlying life choices, like what you eat, how you sleep, how much stress, and certain body indicators to come up with a fix that has little or no side effects, as long as you are willing to do your part.

The connection between the esophagus and the stomach is surrounded by a flap called the lower esophageal sphincter, which prevents acid from going up from the stomach into the esophagus. If this smooth muscle does not function well or the pressure in the stomach suddenly goes up, acid can go up to the esophagus, causing irritation of its membrane, even Barretts Syndrome, which in rare cases can lead to cancer.

Symptoms: heartburn, stomach pain, excess salivation, shortness of breath, difficult or painful swallowing, nausea, vomiting, lightheadedness, sudden blood pressure drop.

What contributes to the acid reflux?

1. Dr. D. Zou and colleagues at Royal Adelaide Hospital in Australia indicates that stomach distension is the major trigger for transient relaxations of the lower esophageal sphincter (LES), the muscle around the connection between the esophagus and the stomach, which can lead to acid reflux.

2. If you eat greasy or protein-rich food, the stomach starts producing acid to digest these foods. The more greasy food one eats, the more acid is produced. Normally, heartburn will not result, but if you combine drinking soda, milk or water at the same time, the pressure in your stomach will increase dramatically, resulting in heartburn or acid reflux.

3. Low serotonin levels and acid reflux: Serotonin is abundantly located in the stomach, the intestinal muscles, and underneath their mucous membranes. It can effectively increase stomach movement to accelerate the emptying of the stomach. As you get older, serotonin levels

may decrease, causing digestion to slow down. Although we eat the same amount of food and drink the same kinds of fluids, we could develop acid reflux. Therefore we need to change our eating habits: eating small meals more frequently and cutting down on greasy and high protein food.

4. Soda and acid reflux: Stomach pressure dramatically increases when food is mixed with fluids, especially soda that has a lot of bubbles. This leads to the opening of the esophageal sphincter. Very often, when people eat salty or spicy food, they become so thirsty right after the meal that they drink too much water, which increases stomach pressure, causing acid reflux.

5. Allergies can cause acid reflux. An allergen not only triggers type-one histamine receptors, which might cause a sneeze or runny nose, but can also trigger a type-two histamine receptors, which stimulate acid secretion in the stomach. In this case, anti-histamine drugs may work well.

6. Stress: When you are constantly in a fight-or-flight condition, your stomach tightens up, increasing stomach pressure. When you drink coffee with cream or sugar right after your meal, acid secretion starts, and increased stomach pressure leads to acid reflux.

7. Overeating: If you eat more than you usually eat, stomach pressure will increase.

8. Obesity: When a person is overweight, there is too much fat around the stomach, pushing on the stomach and increasing pressure. Furthermore, hormone changes in overweight people, causing weaker muscles. According to an article in *The International Journal of Epidemiology* in 2003, overweight people are three times more likely to develop heartburn, compared to the norm.

9. Hiatal Hernia: If you never exercise, not only do your arm and leg muscles become weak, but also your esophagus sphincter muscle, especially as you age. If you take muscle relaxants for a nervous bladder, an estrogen blocker, or Lipitor, you are more prone to develop hiatal hernia, in which the stomach will bulge into the upper chest cavity through the diaphragm, leading to more frequent acid reflux.

10. Strong coffee and tea: Strong coffee will put you in a fight or flight condition: your stomach becomes a fist, the pressure increases. Strong tea slows down your stomach and intestinal movement, so the food stays for a longer time, causing indigestion and increased stomach pressure. Fermented food will produce excessive gas, which will open the esophagus sphincter. If you drink tea without sugar or milk, you will not have a strong appetite, because tea slows down your digestion. Therefore, tea drinkers tend to be on the skinny side. The best tea

drinking time is two hours after your meal, so that you will not have indigestion.

11. Raw tomatoes and onions: Some people cannot digest those foods well, causing acid reflux, or they may be allergic to them. I found out that if you steam tomatoes, you might not have acid reflux.

12. Too much sugar slows down stomach movement. That is why feeding your child ice cream first will cause him/her not to eat the main course. If you feed children ice cream afterwards, they will end up having indigestion.

13. Bubbling water, which has a lot of $CO2$, producing extra H^+ and also increasing stomach pressure.

14. Lack of physical work: Many of us now spend too much time sitting, while driving, working at the computer, or playing video games; this slows down stomach movement and causes indigestion.

15. Eating too fast: We rush through our meals, sometimes standing up, sometimes driving the car, sometimes in a meeting. As a result of not chewing enough, food is not chopped into small enough pieces and mixed thoroughly with saliva. We shouldn't be surprised to end up with indigestion, bloating and gas. As your stomach pressure increases, guess where that pressure goes.

16. Certain medications: morphine, meperidine, nitrate heart medications, and Fosamax, can lead to heartburn, gas, and reflux.

17. Spicy food, sweets, alcohol, and chocolate can relax the muscle around the esophagus. If you have acid reflux currently, try to avoid these triggers until the symptoms are completely gone. Then you can reintroduce those foods in small quantities, twice a week.

18. Autoimmune diseases such as scleroderma, in which the sphincter loses its ability to constrict during eating. Balancing your immune function can help you avoid this life threatening disease.

19. Pregnant women have a very high progesterone level, which relaxes their uterus muscle as well as the lower esophageal sphincter.

20. Late dinner: If you have your dinner around 8pm, it is very likely that you will end up having indigestion. The undigested food can produce gas and increase stomach pressure. It is recommended to go to bed at least 3 hours after dinner.

21. Eating crackers can cause slight laceration of the esophagus, stomach and lower esophageal sphincter. If you eat spicy food or other triggering foods afterwards, you may have a burning sensation.

22. Wearing tight clothing can increase stomach pressure.

Anti-acid Medication:

Many people take anti-acid medications, which strongly inhibit the secretion of acid in the stomach. Do you know that protein needs to be broken down into amino acids in a very acidic environment in order to be effectively absorbed? If we do not have enough acid, the resulting indigestion of protein can produce a deficiency of vitamin B12 and B6, causing anemia, possibly an imbalance of the immune system and nervous system and other serious medical conditions. Medications can resolve the problem temporarily, but we must find the root cause to each health issue so that we can avoid taking medications for too long.

When a person with anxiety disorder takes anti-acid medication for too long, he/she can develop frequent panic attacks due to a Vitamin B deficiency associated with an unhealthy nervous system. Such people cannot drive across a bridge or be in a meeting in a closed room because their nerves become so unstable that lowered oxygen in a closed area or changing their body position suddenly can make their heart beat faster, palms become sweatier, and breathing becomes difficult. When a person has allergies, taking anti-acid medication will decrease the secretion of stomach acid, so that nuts and other protein cannot be digested thoroughly. The undigested protein molecules slip through the intestinal blood vessels, causing worse allergic reactions.

In 2005, E. Untersmayr èt al. of the Center of Physiology at the Medical University of Vienna, Austria, published an article in the *Journal of Allergy Clinical Immunology* about the effects of gastric digestion on codfish-related allergies. Using animal models, codfish extract was mixed with stomach solutions having pH values ranging from 1.25 to 5.0. Codfish proteins degraded within 1 minute under normal stomach conditions. A marginal pH shift from 2.5 to 2.75 completely abrogated the digestion of codfish protein.

When protein is not broken down into smaller molecules, its ability to cause allergies increases 10,000 times, as evaluated on the basis of histamine release. Therefore, impairment of digestion might lower the threshold level of a food allergen in sensitized people. This research beautifully correlates with recent findings that introducing adult food to babies too early and eating too many hamburgers may be associated with the increased incidence of food allergies in the United States. In Chinese medicine, we think that indigestion is the major cause of many kinds of illness, allergies included.

My case study for Acid Reflux:

Casey Ling and I were friends at school. We were both undergraduates at Beijing University of Chinese Medicine. We shared a dorm room for a year and got to know each other that way. We spent time together mostly in silence since we had a common passion to study, read and pursue the healing arts both technically and philosophically. I lost touch with her after graduation, since we did our residencies at different hospitals. She found me again halfway round the world by accident when looking on- line for someone to treat her hives.

She surprised me by calling and giving her married name when making the appointment. I didn't recognize her voice since I was out on my daily walk, and the wind was in my ear when my office redirected her call to my mobile phone.

I remembered her at first glimpse as she hesitantly opened the door to my clinic. When she first came to see me, she was 40 years old. As I did my intake interview, it occurred to me that there was much I didn't know about her when we were friends way back then. For example, she had had hives since childhood. Anti-histamine medication or prednisone had not helped her hives in the past. She used to take the patent herb, Fang Feng Tong Sheng, for a few days, which helped temporarily; the rashes would be gone for a couple of months. Whenever she didn't get enough sleep or was under stress for a period of time, her rashes would show up again. I knew none of this then.

Casey had a bad case of hives. I mention here, in some detail, how I treated her hives. I do that because acid reflux and hives often have the same root causes from a Chinese Medicine standpoint. She had acid reflux most of the time when she had hives, but it was of secondary importance to her because her hives were on display for all to see.

Each time she got pregnant, she tended to get hives. When she was doing her residency in China, one of the doctors there had the same problem and told her to try some H_2 histamine receptor blocker, which is used to treat acid reflux and stomach ulcers. It worked for her hives, but she was afraid that long-term usage of the drug could damage her liver function.

She told me that after she had her first child, her hives returned once or twice a year. She never had heartburn, but sometimes she experienced bloating and indigestion after eating greasy food. For the previous 3 years, she had worked 7 days a week and had not gotten enough sleep most of the time. Moreover, she had been eating dinner very late, just two hours before going to sleep. I know this problem; I often work 7 days a week, and I have had to force myself to take time off. I find that, when I take a break, many problems go away, some physical, some emotional. The big benefit for me is an increase in my ability to find creative solutions to difficult problems that involve seemingly different areas of thought. You have to give yourself a break even when the pressure is on... ESPECIALLY WHEN THE PRESSURE IS ON!!

In August 2003, after Casey drank two small glasses of red wine and ate more than usual at her students' graduation party, her hives started again and lasted for almost 10 months. In addition, after a couple of months, she developed nausea and heartburn. Whenever the heartburn started, her blood pressure would drop, and she would feel extremely tired and unable to focus on anything. She tried doxypin, prilosec, an anti-histamine medication, but nothing seemed to help. What could this be?

At one time, the rashes were so severe that her physician gave her cortisone shots twice a week. Although the rashes would disappear for a day after the shot, they came back even worse the next day.

An abdominal CAT scan was normal. A blood test for food allergies came back negative. Her rashes were often gone during the daytime, but every morning some part of her body would be swollen. One winter morning, her eyes and lips were so swollen that she could not see and had to cancel her class at school. She noticed that cold, heat, wind, hunger, and anxiety all aggravated her hives. Casey needed help, and no solution was forthcoming.

As I thought further, it became apparent that her heartburn was being triggered by strong coffee, sweets and greasy and spicy food. Doing my exam, I found that, at first, her pulse was slippery and slightly wiry, but, after a couple of months, it was fine and weak. Palpitation exams revealed that the rashes felt warm. Stomach discomfort was relieved when pressure was applied to the abdominal area. Her tongue was dry with a red tip, red dots, and transverse cracks on the front third. At the back, there was a slightly thick coating. These various components of my exam indicated to me that she has blocked heat in the upper and middle burner.

Overall, the patient was fairly healthy. Her cheeks looked red, and her skin was quite dry. Her hives could appear at any place on the body at any time. After two months of struggling with her hives using medications that did not seem to help, she got two cortisone shots and gained 5 pounds within a week. Rather than continuing to gain weight, she decided to take herbs and get acupuncture two or three times a week.

Two formulas were used: one specific to the hives, the other for heartburn and digestive issues.

For the hives, based on Qing Ying Tang:

Formula: Sheng Di 10g, Dan Pi 10g, Xuan Shen 15g, Mai Dong 10g, Jin Yin Hua 6g, Lian Qiao 6g, Ban Xia 10g, Chi Shao 15g, Zhi Gan Cao 6g, Chan Yi 6g, Fu Ping 10g, Fu Ling 12g.

For acid reflux and digestive issues:

Formula: Chai Hu 10g, Chi Shao 10g, Bai Shao 10g, Gui Zhi 10g, Zhi Qiao6g, Ban Xia 10g, Zhi Gan Cao 10g, Chuan Xong 6g, Xiang Fu 10g, and Wa Leng Zi 10g.

Casey took the first formula in the mornings and evenings and the second formula during the daytime, especially right before she felt, based on previous experience that her acid reflux might start.

Acupuncture twice a week consisted of the points: SP10, ST36, LI4, LI11, UB44, CV14, Bai Chong Wuo, TW5, UB17, PC7.

Casey reported that 20 minutes after drinking the second herbal formula, she felt the acid reflux go away. The itchiness disappeared within half an hour of taking the first herbal formula first thing in the morning, so I felt I had correctly diagnosed the root of her problems.

I always think about my patients' whole lifestyle so I gave Casey some nutritional suggestions: I said, "Casey, you must avoid greasy and spicy foods, coffee, seafood, nuts, red wine and other kinds of alcohol." She looked at me as if I had given her a severe punishment. "How can I stop drinking wine and eating good food? I love those things." So I explained that she should stop eating those foods while she still has the hives and acid reflux; once the symptoms are completely gone, she can reintroduce those food in small amounts slowly and find the right amounts her body can digest thoroughly. That in itself will be her motivation. Getting to feel better motivates! I finished my advice by telling her to eat dinner before 7 PM and reduce her meat intake in the evening. Also, she should avoid running in cold, windy weather, try to reduce work hours, and get enough sleep. Enough sleep makes her adrenal gland produce optimal levels of cortisol, an anti-allergy hormone.

Casey's hives and acid reflux were much better after 3 months of herbs. After another 3 months, they were completely gone and have not come back for about three years. If she drinks too much coffee before her period, she still feels an itchy sensation, and her face turns red, or some red patches appear. If she stops drinking coffee and takes herbs for a week, her symptoms disappear.

Scientific evidence about acupuncture and acid reflux:

Dr. D. Zou and colleagues at Royal Adelaide Hospital in Australia used acupuncture to treat 14 healthy volunteers at the PC6 (2 cun above transverse crease of wrist, between tendons of medial palmaris longus and medial flexor radialis) and a sham point on the hip, in a randomized order on the same day. The results showed that electrical acupoint stimulation at the PC6 decreased the rate of lower esophageal sphincter relaxations by approximately 40%, from a median of 6 per hour to 3.5 per hour. Acupoint stimulation had no effect on the basal lower esophageal sphincter tone.

Doctors at the University of Rochester School of Medicine and Dentistry found that electrical acupuncture can not only reduce the basal acid secretion in dogs, but it can also inhibit meal-stimulated acid secretion in dogs through increased levels somatostatin.

Dr. G.C. Sugai et al. of the Department of Orthopedics and Traumatology at the Universidade Federal de Sao Paulo of Brazil investigated how serotonin plays an important role in mediating the effects of acupuncture on gastric emptying in rats. They used a type of glass bead flow to measure the stomach-emptying speed. Electrical acupuncture on ST36 (4 finger-breadth distal to external knee eye in the depression lateral to the patellar ligament, 1 finger breadth lateral to the crest of the tibia) and SP6 (4 finger-breadth superior to medial malleolus) or moxibustion (burning a certain kind of herb called mugwort) above the abdominal points, CV10 (on the midline of the abdomen, 2 inches above the umbilicus) increased the flow of glass beads in the rat's stomach, indicating that acupuncture can speed up stomach movement. After they applied a serotonin receptor blocker, this effect was abolished.

How you can deal with acid reflux:

1. Separate fluid and food: drink water half an hour before your food, especially if you are going to eat in a restaurant. While you are waiting for your food, you can drink some lukewarm or room temperature water to prepare your stomach for greasy and salty food.

Please do not drink any ice-cold water, which constricts the stomach membrane blood vessels, causing dysfunction of your enzymes. The digestive enzymes work best at certain temperatures. That is why in old China, whenever a child had indigestion, parents would give him/her a warm pad. During my residency training, the only time I asked a patient to drink ice-cold water was when he/she had bleeding in the digestive system.

2. Do not drink strong coffee or tea right after your meal or on an empty stomach. Light tea or coffee is better served between meals.

3. If you have allergies, you need to find out what food triggers acid reflux. Nuts, raw tomatoes, and raw onions can do the trick.

4. Eat half an apple before or two hours after your meal. Certain enzymes in the apple help your stomach digest greasy food. That is why some people have told me that, after they eat an apple, they feel hungry two hours later. However, if you eat an apple right after your meal, the effect is not the same.

5. Raw cucumbers can also help digestion to clear up the acid reflux.

6. Do not drink milk with your food. Drink it between meals. Lactose causes slow digestion, bloating and gas, especially for Asians.

7. Adding barley or Daikon into your soup will help your digestion. You can also boil your meat with Daikon to help digest the meat protein and oil.

8. If you want to have optimal health, always eat 80% full. In a village in Yun Nan province of China, there are many 100-year-old people. One of the reasons for leading their long and happy lives is that they do not eat too much.

9. Sit down and chew each mouthful of food at least twenty times so that you can enjoy and digest the food slowly. In this way, we can eat less food because our brain has the time to process the full sensation.

10. If you eat a very greasy meal, and you feel you may get acid reflux, do not drink any fluids for the next two hours, and try to walk but not run for half an hour or an hour. Walking increases your stomach movement, so that your stomach can digest food faster, and the food will not stay in your stomach, causing stomach pressure to go up. In 1960, China experienced a very difficult time after Chairman Mao broke up China's relationship with the Soviet Union. Everybody was assigned a very small amount of food each day for two to three years, so their digestion became weaker. When a holiday came, people ate too much and drank water afterwards. Their stomachs became so much enlarged that they could hardly move, and some people died of overeating. Never keep eating until you feel full if you want to be healthy.

Chinese Herbal medicine and acupuncture for acid reflux:

Chinese herbs and acupuncture can improve your digestion and speed up the emptying of your stomach; certain herbs can absorb the acid quickly for quick relief, and most of herbs can be used to treat the root cause according to the diagnosis.

1. Stomach heat and deficiency of spleen:

Symptoms: always feeling hungry, bad breath, constipation, bloating and gas after eating, easily developing rashes, red tip of nose, red tongue with yellow thick coating, pulse: slippery.

Formula: Huang Lian 6g, Sheng Di 9g, Sheng Da Huan 6g, Dang Gui 9g, Wa Leng Zi 10g, Zhi Zi 6g, Zhi Gan Cao 6g, Sheng Hang Qi 9g, Fu ling 12g.

People with this diagnosis always have a good appetite, but they tend to eat too much. Because their spleen is overloaded, food is not digested properly. The undigested food produces a heat toxin in their stomach, causing acid reflux. In this formula, we not only strengthen spleen function to improve digestion but also clear the stomach heat so that the person does not eat too much.

Acupuncture points:

ST36: On the anterior aspect of the lower leg, 3 cun below the depression lateral to the patella ligament, one finger-breadth (middle finger) from the anterior crest of the tibia. Insert needle with 30^0 angle toward ST37 with 2 inches needle.

ST37: On the anterior aspect of the lower leg, 6 cun below the depression lateral to the patella ligament, one finger-breadth (middle finger) from the anterior crest of the tibia.

ST38: On the anterior aspect of the lower leg, 8 cun below the depression lateral to the patella ligament, one finger-breadth (middle finger) from the anterior crest of the tibia.

CV10: On the anterior median line of the upper abdomen, 2.0 cun above the umbilicus.

2. Spleen deficiency with phlegm

Symptoms: a tendency to be overweight, swelling of ankles or hands, phlegm in the throat, diarrhea, sleeping more than 8 hours, but still feeling tired and, pale complexion.

Formula: Dang Sheng 9g, Fu Ling 20g, Jiang Ban Xia 6g, Chen Pi 6g, Zhi Gan Cao 6g, Wa Leng Zi 15g, Chao Mai Ya 15g, Cang Zhu 6g.

Acupuncture and acupressure points:

SP9: On the medial aspect of the lower leg, in the depression of the lower border of the medial condyle of the tibia.

CV11: On the anterior median line of the upper abdomen, 3.0 cun above the umbilicus.

PC6: On the palmar aspect of the forearm, 2 cun above the transverse crease of the wrist, between the tendons of m. palmaris longus and m. flexor carpi radialis.

Tian Huang Fu Xue: 3 inches directly below SP9

3. Liver Qi insulting spleen:

Symptoms: irritability, mood swing, acid reflux gets worse if patient gets stressed or angry.

Formula: Chai Hu 10g, Chi Shao 10g, Bai Shao 10g, Zhi Qiao 6g, Ban Xia 10g, Zhi Gan Cao10g, Chuan Xiong 6g, Xiang Fu 10g, Wa Leng Zi 15g, Chuan Lian Zi 6g.

Acupressure points for self-healing:

CV6 (Qi Hai): On the anterior median line of the lower abdomen, 1.5 cun below the umbilicus.

Liv6 (Zhong Du): On the medial aspect of the lower leg, 7 cun above the tip of the medial malleolus, on the middle of the medial aspect of the tibia.

CV16 (Zhong Ting): On the anterior median line of the chest, at the level of the 5th intercostal space, near the xiphisternal synchondroses.

34

CV13: On the anterior median line of the upper abdomen, 5.0 cun above the umbilicus

Chapter Three

Insomnia

According to a report from the 2002 edition of *Brain Facts*, a publication of the Society for Neuroscience, sleep disorders affect up to 70 million people in the United States and cost about $100 billion each year in accidents, medical bills, and loss of work. In the theory of Chinese medicine, a healthy life is based on the balance of Yin and Yang. During the daytime, Yang is dominant, and we are awake; Yin is dominant at night, and we fall asleep. If Yang, the energy, cannot go inside of our body, we will have difficulty sleeping. When we reach a certain age, our Yin level will start decreasing, so we must change our life style accordingly to achieve a new balance between the Yin and Yang. For instance, we should avoid alcohol and coffee consumption, late parties, and we should go to bed at a fixed time.

What are the cycles of our sleep?

Sleep follows a regular cycle each night. There are two basic forms of sleep: rapid eye movement (REM) sleep and non-REM

(NREM) sleep. Infants spend about 50% of their sleep time in NREM and 50% in REM sleep. Adults spend about 20% of their sleep time in REM and 80% in NREM sleep. Elderly people spend less than 15% of their sleep time in REM sleep. There is a large variation in total sleep time and the percentage of REM and NREM sleep among individuals.

NREM sleep can be divided into 4 stages, 1, 2, 3 and 4, each with different brain electrical activity patterns. Stages 3 and 4 are called slow wave sleep (SWS), or deep sleep, during which the brain has fewer activities. Research has shown dramatic decreases in blood flow to certain areas of the brain during deep sleep as compared to wakefulness. While we are asleep, our brains are on a bit of a "roller coaster ride" through different stages of sleep. As we drift off to sleep, we enter stage 1 sleep. After a few minutes, we enter stage 2 sleep, and then stage 3, and then stage 4. Next it's back up the steps again: stage 3, and then stage 2, followed by a period of REM sleep. The cycle then resumes.

During an 8-hour period of sleep, the brain cycles through these stages about 4-5 times, which means we go through one cycle every two hours. During REM sleep, our eyes move quickly, our breath becomes irregular and accelerated, our blood pressure rises, and our muscles lose their tone (paralysis); our brain remains highly active, however. The electrical activity in the brain during REM sleep is similar to that recorded during wakefulness. REM sleep is usually associated with dreams. Often when people wake up from REM sleep, they will say that they were just dreaming. The inactivity of our muscles during REM sleep prevents us from acting out our dreams. REM sleep is important for memory and learning.

Longer periods of slow wave (deep) sleep (SWS) occur in the first part of the night, primarily in the first two sleep cycles (roughly 3 hours). Children and young adults have more total SWS in a night than older adults, so they are more likely to wake up during SWS sleep. On the other hand, the elderly may not reach deep sleep (stage 3 and 4) at all for many nights. The highest arousal thresholds are observed in deep sleep. One will typically feel groggier when awakened from these stages. People awakened from deep sleep will have slightly impaired mental performances for a period of up to 30 minutes in cognitive tests compared to those awakened from other stages. When people are deprived of deep sleep for a while, they will have more deep sleep at a later time to compensate, suggesting that there is more of a "need" for it relative to the other stages.

Factors that influence our sleep cycles:

1. Serotonin, a neurotransmitter, can influence both REM and NREM sleep. Generally, serotonin enhances stages 3 and 4 (deep sleep) but inhibits REM sleep. If people are depressed and lack serotonin, they may reach REM sleep more quickly, resulting in an increase in the REM percentage of total sleep and a significantly longer first REM period. At

the same time, serotonin deficiency may cause a decrease in the deep sleep time, during which the brain has less activity. People often wake up during the REM stage, feeling depressed and exhausted mentally because the brain did not get enough rest from deep sleep.

Selective serotonin reuptake inhibitors can reduce REM in mammals and birds. In a matched control study in 2004, Winkelman and James at the Sleep Health Center of Harvard Medical School observed that patients taking serotonergic antidepressants had more muscle activity during REM than the control group. Since people taking serotonergic antidepressants cannot relax their muscles completely during REM sleep, they may act out their dreams. Dr. Ulrich Voderholzer and colleagues in the Department of Psychiatry and Psychotherapy of the University Hospital of Freiburg, Germany, investigated how a low serotonin level, induced by depletion of tryptophan, from which serotonin is made, influenced sleep patterns. They noticed an increase in the number of waking periods and the amount of waking time when blood serotonin was low, along with an increase in the overall density of REM sleep. Often, when people use serotonin reuptake blockers to treat depression, they fall asleep more easily and wake up less often but still feel tired and foggy-headed. This may result from the disproportional enhancement of deep sleep and reduction of REM sleep by too much serotonin.

2. Acetylcholine: acetylcholine levels are high during waking and REM stages and low during slow wave sleep periods. Dr. Anne E. Power of the University of California at Irvine suggests that acetylcholine regulates the flow of information between the hippocampus and the neocortex, which is important for effective long-term memory consolidation. Any medication influencing acetylcholine levels may potentially interrupt REM and SWS sleep.

3. Adrenaline: High adrenaline can also disturb sleep patterns. If you have too much adrenaline, your muscles cannot completely relax during REM sleep and your legs or arms may move around. This condition is called restless leg syndrome (RLS), which produces an intense, irresistible urge to move the legs because of creeping, crawling, tingling, and burning sensations. Arthur Walters and David Rye, Professor of Neurology at Emory University School of Medicine, says that periodic limb movements disorder (PLMS), seen in most restless leg syndrome patients, are associated with the increased activity of sympathetic nervous system. Anything that can dramatically increase your adrenaline release, such as coffee, overexcitement, high sugar intake, or a medication that interrupts the metabolism of adrenaline, can potentially interrupt your sleep.

4. Melatonin (N-acetyl-5-methoxytryptamine) is a hormone produced by the pineal gland in the brain in response to darkness. Melatonin becomes available when tryptophan is converted to serotonin

and then reconfigured to melatonin in the pineal gland. There is a very close relationship between serotonin and melatonin, and anything that affects serotonin or melatonin can change one's sleep pattern. Melatonin levels in the blood are low during the day, with peak levels occurring at 2-4 AM. Many lines of research indicate that melatonin deficiency may play a key role in anxiety-associated insomnia.

5. Alcohol: The duration of slow wave sleep (deep sleep) can be lengthened by the ingestion of alcohol. In this scenario, total sleep time is often unaffected because of circadian rhythms and/or a person's alarm clock and early morning obligations. This increase of deep sleep can lead to delayed REM onset and a decrease in REM sleep. Alcoholics usually wake up feeling depressed and groggy for the whole morning.

6. The balance of our autonomic nervous systems: sympathetic and parasympathetic activities have to be balanced during the day and night. During daytime, when we are thinking and working, the sympathetic nervous system predominates. At night, the parasympathetic nervous system becomes more active than the sympathetic as we digest food and relax, as our immune system rejuvenates, and as different kinds of tissues repair themselves. When you are exposed to acute stress, adrenaline will be present at relatively high concentrations in your blood circulation; this can stimulate your sympathetic nervous system, causing insomnia. When you talk too much, think too much, or drink too much caffeine, you also over-

stimulate your sympathetic nervous system, which will interrupt your sleep. You will either have difficulty falling asleep or wake up in the middle of the night.

7. β-endorphin and insomnia: Have you ever experienced difficulty sleeping after intensive pre-bedtime exercises? You feel very energetic after the exercise and cannot fall asleep until after midnight. Intensive exercise not only stimulates the release of adrenaline but also of ß-endorphin. Therefore, you should avoid intensive exercises starting 3 hours before you want to go to sleep.

8. Menopausal hormone changes: During menopause, women stop ovulating, and the progesterone levels in their bodies decrease dramatically. Progesterone has a soothing effect and makes sleep deeper and sounder. With a reduced progesterone level, the nervous system becomes more sensitive to external changes. After menopause, there are two sources of progesterone: fat tissue and the adrenal gland. If you are too skinny or you're under stress, then your adrenal gland function will be compromised, and your sleep pattern will change even though you were a good sleeper before. Clinically, slightly heavier people sleep better than very thin people with more adaptability to environmental changes.

How Acupuncture treats insomnia

Hormones and the autonomic nervous system have to be balanced in order to initiate and maintain sleep. Many studies have shown that acupuncture treatments can help maintain the balance of biological chemicals in the central nervous system and promote the recovery of homeostasis.

Acupuncture can help your body produce more melatonin:

In an article published in the *Journal of Neuropsychiatry and Clinical Neuroscience*, Spence et al. explored the relationship between melatonin and acupuncture treatments. They observed a significant increase in endogenous melatonin secretion in all of the 18 patients suffering from severe insomnia who were given acupuncture treatments twice a week for 5 weeks. Records of electrical and muscular states during the entire sleeping time indicated that, after acupuncture treatments, the patients took less time to fall asleep, had fewer occasions of waking up during sleep, and experienced increased total sleep time and deep sleep time. Anxiety, depression, and fatigue were also decreased. Interestingly, alertness in the morning was reduced as well. In my acupuncture practice, I noticed that people who sleep more than 8 to 10 hours tend to be drowsier in the morning than people who sleep only 6 to 7 hours. This phenomenon may explain why many people need to drink coffee before they hit the road. People with good sleep, however, can function better later on without anxiety and without a sudden decrease of energy in the early afternoon.

Acupuncture can improve blood flow to improve sleep quality

Hecht and his colleagues studied the relationship between the blood flow to the brain and insomnia. They noted that an insufficient blood flow to the brain could lead to low sugar levels and spontaneous waking from sleep. Dr. Omura explored the effects of blood flow to the brain on the dysfunctions of various organs. When blood pressure in the head was very low (less than 30 mmHg on both sides), a majority of the subjects experienced sleep disturbances: mainly insomnia but sometimes excessive-sleepiness, difficulty concentrating, forgetfulness of recent events, and various degrees of irritability. Even with normal or higher arm blood pressure, one can still have low blood pressure in one's head. It has been reported that electro-acupuncture stimulation of the points ST36 and GB20 (just inferior to occipital bone, between the trapezius and sternocleidomastoid attachments) can treat insomnia by increasing the blood flow to the brain.

Acupuncture can decrease effects of aging:

The weakening of parasympathetic function results in the familiar signs of aging, including increased and irregular heartbeats, constipation, insomnia, erectile dysfunction, fluid retention, and systematic inflammation. These consequences may in turn contribute to many of the common diseases associated with aging, including Type-II diabetes, Alzheimer's, arteriosclerosis, and cancer. The maintenance and restoration of parasympathetic function may boost the functions of the internal organs and slow the aging process. Acupuncture generally enhances the parasympathetic nervous system.

Acupuncture can reduce pain:

Meltzer at the Children's Hospital of Philadelphia studied the effects of chronic pain on the sleep patterns of adolescents. He found no difference between the pain group and the healthy control group in total sleep time and bedtime. However, the group with chronic pain reported significantly longer sleep onset latency, more frequent night waking, later wake times in the morning, and more symptoms of daytime sleepiness. Acupuncture has a very good analgesic effect and can thereby help people with pain improve their sleep quality.

Acupuncture can reduce stress hormones to treat insomnia

When we are under chronic stress, such as over-thinking and overworking, our body produces more cortisol to keep us alert during the daytime. When we are under acute stress, such as a fight-or-flight condition, our body produces more epinephrine (adrenaline) and norepinephrine. These two stress hormones deeply affect our sleep quality. Vgontzas and colleagues at the Pennsylvania State University assessed the association of chronic insomnia with the activity of the stress system. They measured the levels of free cortisol, norepinephrine, and growth hormone in the urine of the participants and found that free cortisol levels correlated positively with total wake time; norepinephrine levels correlated positively with the duration of stage 1 sleep but negatively with the duration of stage 3 and 4 (deep) sleep. Both branches of the stress system (the adrenal gland and the sympathetic nervous system) are accountable for the sleep disturbances in chronic insomnia. When we are stressed, our sleep is much lighter, so we wake up more frequently. Acupuncture can lower stress hormone levels, thereby reducing wake time and increasing deep sleep time. It is well known that cortisone can influence sleep when we receive a hydrocortisone shot.

Different acupuncture styles and manipulations affect the levels of different chemicals such as ß-endorphin, serotonin, cortisol, dopamine, and GABA. To balance the chemicals, the right treatment methods have to be implemented. Very strong electro-acupuncture stimulation before bedtime may lead to temporary insomnia. After a long duration of electro-acupuncture, some patients report that they have difficulty sleeping the first night but that they could still function very well the next day. The duration and timing of electrical stimulation should be fine-tuned to fit each individual's situation.

In conclusion, NREM and REM sleep must be in balance. NREM sleep relaxes us mentally, and REM sleep relaxes our muscles. Too much REM sleep is associated with depression, whereas too much NREM sleep leads to drowsiness because the brain is in deep relaxation. We need the right amounts of both kinds of sleep. By optimizing the production and metabolism of chemicals that affect sleep, acupuncture can maintain the appropriate sleep pattern and duration.

How to prevent insomnia

1. Bathing in a hot tub can dilate the blood vessels on your body's surface to induce relaxation and deeper sleep.

2. Intense, prolonged exercise during the daytime can help increase deep sleep. However, if exercise is performed too close to bedtime, it may delay the onset of sleep by increasing the secretion of adrenaline.

3. Balance the activity of the nervous system by practicing meditation, yoga, tai ji, qi gong, and stretching exercises two hours before you go to bed.

4. Change sleep-disturbing habits such as watching television in bed or keeping an irregular bedtime schedule.

5. Avoid the use of stimulants and depressants such as tobacco, caffeine, and alcohol within 6 hours of your bedtime. The best time to drink coffee is in the morning because some people, especially women, cannot clear up the caffeine in their bodies within 16 hours.

6. Engage in regular physical activities, especially yoga and Pilates, which enhance parasympathetic function.

7. Check all of your medications with your doctor to see whether they affect your sleep; you may be able to adjust your prescriptions or schedule to avoid creating sleep problems. Many people take anti-anxiety medications, for which one of the side effects is insomnia. Combining acupuncture with the lowest possible dosage of the medication can prevent this side effect, because acupuncture stimulates your own body to optimize hormone levels.

8. Reserve the bed for sleeping and sexual activity only.

9. Don't stay in bed longer than 8 hours, and try to avoid taking long naps.

10. Use the evening hours for settling down; avoid challenging activities within 2 hours of bedtime. Talking on the phone after 8 PM will disturb your sleep. If you need to make a phone call, do it right after an early dinner.

11. Eat meals at regularly scheduled times, and eliminate late dinners and bedtime snacks, because a full stomach and high blood sugar can keep you awake.

12. Once you are in bed, relax from head to toe, and guide your mind towards pleasant thoughts. Reading novels in your bed may help your sleep, but many people wake up earlier or cannot fall asleep because the exciting stories may stimulate different parts of your brain.

13. Get plenty of sunlight outdoors, particularly later in the afternoon.

14. Keep your bedroom quiet, dark, and cool. Try using a sleep mask and earplugs to help you sleep.

15. Restrict nighttime liquid consumption to reduce the need to get up to urinate, but don't go to bed thirsty.

16. Avoid uneven noises (sometimes a steady "white noise" such as a running fan can help), being too hot or too cold, and the bright lights of a television and/or a computer screen during the late afternoon, evening, or at night, which may reduce your melatonin secretion.

If you try all of the above, and your sleep is still not good, try taking some Chinese herbs to balance your hormone levels. Chinese herbal medicines are multi-target and produce hardly any drowsiness or addiction. However, it will take one to six months to reestablish a healthy sleep cycle. People who are extremely sensitive to sleeping pills usually respond better to herbs.

For chronic sleep disorders, get acupuncture 3 times a week for 10 treatments, then twice a week for another 10 treatments, followed by once a week for 10 more treatments if necessary. Acupuncture once a week is not enough to correct the problems unless you combine it with herbal medicines.

Case Study

This is the only time I will use myself as an example of case study. I am doing this because I have had serious sleep problems during my life. I have sometimes treated myself, and sometimes I have had treatment from my fellow professionals. Hopefully, the benefit for the reader in having me tell the story is that I know much more about symptoms and causality because I am a practitioner and patient in one. So read on, and you decide.

I have been a light sleeper ever since I was a child. When I was a teenager, I would often wake up in the middle of the night, planning the next day's activities. I would think about a big test or a difficult social situation I had gotten into or, on a rare occasion, the boy I really liked. After 2 to 3 hours, I would finally fall back to sleep. When I was in college, I shared a room with six other girls. I developed a routine that would help me sleep: I would first soak my feet in hot water, then recite some boring Chinese poem after I reviewed all my medical class notes, making sure to go to bed before 10:30 PM. I would sleep 7 to 8 hours when I followed this routine. On some occasions, I could not fall asleep until 4 or 5 AM, for example, when I danced with loud, crazy, music with my classmates, celebrating New Year's Eve. However, during the next night, I could easily sleep 7 or 8 hours to make up the lost time. During my internship year, I had to take a night shift every three days. When I was on the night shift, I used to check all my patients after dinner time, and then check them again around 10 PM. If most of the patients were stable, I would lie down in my working room reading some boring medical journal and doze off for a few hours. In my deep mind, I was worrying about those patients in their critical conditions, so a very light noise would wake me up, and I would stay up for the rest of the night, listening to patients going back and forth to the bathroom. The next day, after I finished my work, I went home, but I still could not sleep during the daytime no matter how tired I was.

I finally got my medical degree and started the 5-year residency. The night shift always disrupted my sleep, and if the night shift was too frequent, I might end up having allergies once or twice a year. I took anti-histamine for my rashes, but I was so drowsy that I would fall asleep as soon as I sat down. One time, I got a prednisone injection, stayed up the whole night, and the next day the rashes came back even worse. In my twenties, I usually could catch up on my sleep once I resumed my normal sleep pattern: go to bed at 11 PM and get up at 6 AM. This indicates that I had a very sensitive nervous system, which responded to changes quickly and profoundly.

In my late twenties and early thirties, I raised two children. I often had to get up in the middle of the night to feed them, and I always had a hard time falling back asleep once I was up. My second child was a very light sleeper and woke up every 2 hours until he was 2 years old. My sleep became so bad that I woke up every 3 hours and took two hours to fall back asleep during my thirties. I was exhausted and always fell asleep on the train ride to work, while at the same time I was teaching, doing research and setting up a new clinical practice. After I had my third child, my sleep became even more interrupted. In the meantime, I started having many other symptoms, including severe irritability and mood swings (one moment I would be happy, and the next minute I would yell at the kids just because they did not start studying as soon as I told them). I also developed intolerance to cold and felt that the bottoms of my feet and the palms of my hands were always hot before my period. My sleep would shorten to merely 4 hours per night a week before my period. Finally, I decided to have acupuncture and take Chinese herbs to fix these problems. Initially, I took herbs every day for 8 months. Later, I changed to taking them just the week before my period. I also started stretching exercises every night an hour before bedtime.

52

You may think this is strange, but I refused to engage in any kind of exciting conversation after 7 PM. Imagine my husband coming in to tell me a funny story, and I say, "oh, no stories, it's too late. He thinks it strange indeed! BUT IT WORKS. I stopped going to late-night parties unless I did not have to work the next day. After 10 months of effort, I could sleep 7 hours without any interruption. Although I occasionally slept only 6 hours, I would catch up a little with 7 hours of sleep the following night. I also noticed that, if I happened to sleep more than 8 hours, I would be drowsy the whole morning unless I had a cup of coffee. After drinking coffee, I would not sleep quite so deeply that night, with my sleep time often dropping to 6 hours.

As I approached 43 years of age, my sleep became more sensitive to daily life changes with a busier schedule and more responsibilities. It got to the point that bright light, noise, or even lack of physical exercise could shorten my deep sleep time. One summer, I changed my daily running habit to walking with my children instead, and I found out that I could not sleep more than 6 hours. If I did not exercise for two days, I would wake up in the middle of the night, and it would be a while before I could fall back to sleep. My mind was clear, and I was not tired the next day, even though I had only slept for 5 hours. This 5 to 6 hour sleep pattern could last weeks, if I did not try to change something. I started a new regimen of exercises: I walked on the treadmill with highest inclination for half an hour 3 hours before bedtime to make myself exhausted physically, and then I would sleep through the night with 7 hours of deep sleep. When I woke up from a seven hour sleep, I noticed that my short term memory was beginning to improve. I was becoming an attentive student of my own minor habits, you see.

I stopped drinking coffee twice a week when I first noticed the sleep changes after I turned to forty-two. I found out that caffeine made my pupils dilate, and I rushed around trying to finish ten things at one time. Moreover, I became anxious and irritable with even just one cup of coffee. In order to stay calm and healthy, I switched to green tea. Two years later, I found out that even tea bothered me! I could not drink green tea after 12 noon. I could sense that my nervous system was so sensitive to stimulants that I could tell the differences between green, black and white tea. Green tea made me super alert, while white tea was more relaxing. When I drank black tea, I was very happy and satisfied. I also noticed that if I drank tea on an empty stomach, my nervous system got so excited that I would be in a hyper-alert condition for the whole day. By the end of the day, I would have a hard time falling asleep, then I would wake up at 4 AM and could not fall back to sleep. When I talked to my fellow acupuncturist, who had hyperthyroid condition, about how tea interrupted my sleep, my friend said: "I had that problem a long time ago."

As I figured out all the factors that influenced my sleep, I arranged all my evening activities to relax and prepare me for a good sleep. While I was traveling in a different time zone, I would take a sleeping pill to get a 7-hour sleep, so that I could give a lecture the next day with a clear mind. One time, I took a sleeping pill for four successive days during a time in China when I had to meet many doctors to discuss my nephew's cancerous condition. I gained 5 pounds within a week. Moreover, after coming back home and stopping this medication, I woke up every two hours. I had to try exercises more during the daytime, acupuncture and Chinese herbs for 4 days to recover my 7-hour sleep. Now I will never take a sleeping pill for more than two days.

Chinese Herbal Formula for insomnia based on different constitution:

1. Liver and heart fire with blood deficiency:

Symptoms: over-thinking, sometimes compulsive thinking, irritability, mood swings, dry skin and eyes, drinking a lot water and still feeling thirsty, good appetite, constipation or sluggish bowel movement, eating a lot of food, high blood pressure, stiff neck or back when exposed to stress, very sensitive to environmental changes and caffeine stimulation, waking up early and having difficulty falling back asleep.

Formula: Chi Hu 12g, Long Gu 20g, Mu Li 20g, Sheng Da Huang 6g, Suan Sao Ren 20g, Chi Shao 20g, Yi Yi Ren 20g, Fu ling 20g, Xiang Fu 12g, Zhi Gan Cao 6g.

2. Heart and kidney cannot communicate with yin deficiency:

Symptoms: lower back and knee weakness and soreness, fatigue, delayed period with small amount of blood, or shortened period interval, night sweats and hot flushes, joint stiffness, dry skin, low endurance for physical activities, heat sensation at the bottoms of the feet or palms of the hands, burning sensation of vagina with frequent urination.

Formula: Niu Zhen Zi 15g, Han Lian Cao 15g, Mai Men Dong 15g, Sheng Di Huang 15g, Shan Yao 20g, Fu ling 20g, Mu Dan Pi 6g, Dan Zhu Ye 12g, Zhi Mu 12g, Zhi Gan Cao 6g.

3. Phlegm and heat accumulating in the middle and upper burner:

Symptoms: phlegmy sensation in the throat, needing to clear the throat all the time, constant post nasal drip, nasal congestion, nausea, thirsty but not wanting to drink water, tendency to develop asthma or sinusitis. Tongue: red with thick yellow coating, Pulse: slippery or forceful.

Formula: Chen Pi 12g, Jiang Ban Xia 12g, Fu Ling 20g, Yi Yi Ren 30g, Zhi Shi 12g, Zhu Ru 12g, Huang Qin 6g, Zhi Gan Cao 6g, Dan Nan Xin 6g.

4. Food stagnation with spleen deficiency:

Symptoms: hungry all the time, bad breath, acid reflux, constipation, foul smelling stool, sluggish bowel movement. Waking up around 4 am, stomach growling, hard to fall asleep. Tongue: red with thick yellow coating at the back, Pulse: slippery.

Formula: Shen Qu 12g, Sheng Shan Zha 12g, Bin Lang 6g, Chao Mai Ya 20g, Zhi Shi 12g, Zhi Gan Cao 6g, Bai Zhu 15g, Fu Ling 20g, Dang Shen12g.

Acupuncture points for insomnia

If you have a digestive issue:

UB21: On the back, 1.5 cun lateral to the lower border of the spinous process of the 12th thoracic vertebra.

HT7: On the wrist, at the ulnar end of the transverse crease of the writs, in the depression on the radial side of the tendon m. flexor carpi ulnaris.

SP6: 3 cun above the medial malleolus, on the posterior border of the medial aspect of the tibia.

If you have irritability and distention of your rib cage:

GV20: At the midpoint of the line connecting the apexes of the two auricles.

PC6: On the palmar aspect of the forearm, 2 cun above the transverse crease of the wrist, between the tendons of m. palmaris longus and m. flexor carpi radialis.

LIV14: On the chest, directly below the nipple, in the 6th intercostal space, 4 cun lateral to the anterior midline.

Si Shen Cong: a group of four points, 1.0 cun respectively anterior, posterior and lateral to the highest point of the head.

If you neck is always tight and your brain lacks blood flow:

UB10: within the posterior hairline, 1.3 cun lateral to the midline, in the depression on the lateral border of m. trapezius.

Head Triangle: from the head of the eyebrow draw two parallel lines, one inch into hairline. These two points form the base of the triangle, and the top point is located on the midline of the head.

Special treatments for insomnia:

Ru Tu (connected with positive electrode), Tai Yang (negative): Electrical stimulation with constant low frequency.

Bai Hui (positive), GB20 (negative) on left or right side: with constant low frequency electrical stimulation.

Hu Bian: in the middle of LI4 and LI3

Chapter Four

High Cholesterol

and Statin

Drugs

High cholesterol must be the most talked about medical condition I know. It seems that many of my friends take statins to treat their cholesterol. This condition silently grows over time in your body. It has no symptoms that you can report to someone. You cannot tell your doctor that you feel like a sticky white substance is coating the inside of your arteries. You have to be told that it exists by a person reporting the results of a blood test. And despite having no symptoms until it is too late (heart attack time), statins are the most prescribed medicines by far. Why is that? How does it happen? What can you do about it besides take these drugs? When you think about it, taking a drug when you have no symptoms is the highest form of faith in

Western Medical Science because from what *you* experience, all you're getting are side effects.

What causes high cholesterol?

Weight: Excess weight may increase your LDL level and losing it may help.

Physical activity/exercise: Regular physical activity may lower triglycerides and raise HDL cholesterol levels.

Age and sex: After menopause, women usually have higher total cholesterol due to decreased hormone and metabolism levels. Generally speaking, aging can cause increased cholesterol level if you do not change your diet just because your body can not clear up the extra cholesterol very efficiently.

Mental stress: Several studies have shown that stress raises blood cholesterol levels over the long term. One way that stress may do this is by affecting your habits. You tend to eat more junk food when you are stressed.

Heredity: Genes may influence how the body processes LDL (bad) cholesterol and could lead to early heart disease.

Functions of cholesterol:

1. Cholesterol is an essential part of all cell membranes, which enables the cell to regulate what enters or leaves them. This regulation is essential to normal cell function. For example, properly working skin cells form a protective coating for our body against infectious diseases and other physical damages.

2. Cholesterol is the raw material for our hormones such as cortisol, DHEA, estrogen, progesterone, and testosterone. In one long-term study, which required all its subjects to eat a low cholesterol diet for more than 5 years, many participants developed low testosterone problems in their later years even though they had lower mortality rates from heart problems.

3. Cholesterol protects the walls of blood vessels. People tend to develop aneurysms if their blood vessels are not strong enough to withstand the pressure from the heart squeezing blood into the aorta, the biggest artery in our body.

4. Cholesterol boosts mental performance. When you try to learn something, new connections called synapses have to form between nerve cells. Glial cells, located among the neurons, produce cholesterol, which, as researchers suggest, plays a critical role in regulating chemical communication between nerve cells and synaptic plasticity. If your body

has an abnormal level of cholesterol, your memory will be compromised, which is why some people develop global amnesia after taking cholesterol drugs, such as Lipitor for many years. To learn more about this topic, please read www.spacedoc.net.

5. Cholesterol provides energy. If you do not have enough fat in your diet, you will be hungry every two hours. Your blood sugar will go up and down, and your brain cells, which need sugar for energy, can suffer from this roller coaster.

6. Cholesterol strengthens muscles. It acts as an important structural component of the nicotinic acetylcholine receptor (a protein which, when combined with neurotransmitters, makes muscles contract) and is vital for the interactions between nerves. Problems of this protein can be associated with Alzheimer's disease, Parkinson's disease, schizophrenia, epilepsy, and addictions to alcohol, nicotine and cocaine. A low fat diet does not necessarily bring down the mortality and morbidity of these detrimental neurodegenerative diseases. I now see more and more people who get Alzheimer's disease in their early fifties and sixties.

7. Cholesterol helps fat digestion because it is a component of bile. If you do not have sufficient bile, you will have diarrhea whenever you eat any kind of fat, even the good oils.

8. Nerve cells do not divide and reproduce like other types of body cells, so they need extra cholesterol to survive longer. If a statin drug such as Lipitor lowers cholesterol levels too much it will cause the early onset of nerve cell death and thus poor memory, depression, and even suicide. A clinical report in the FDA database, for example, indicated that statin drugs might induce subclinical yet important memory loss.

9. Cholesterol helps the body absorb fat-soluble vitamins such as vitamins A, E, and K. Even if you take many kinds of dietary supplements, if your body cannot absorb them well, the deficiency of the above vitamins will cause bleeding and blood clots as well as vision problems.

Forms of Cholesterol:

HDL: High-Density Lipoprotein is the good form of cholesterol.

LDL: Low-Density Lipoprotein is the bad form of cholesterol.

As we get older, our cholesterol levels naturally increase slightly because our cholesterol clearing system no longer functions as efficiently as it did when we were younger. Therefore, we ought to change our diet. However, because our own bodies produce 80% of our cholesterol, eating fat does not necessarily result in a higher cholesterol level.

What can cause your total cholesterol level to go up?

1. Insufficient Intake of Vegetables.

2. Declining enzyme function: Older people have less efficient enzymes to clear up cholesterol than younger ones. Therefore, we need to change our diets or cut our food portions accordingly as we age.

3. Drinking wine every evening: Although red wine increases your HDL (good cholesterol), it also raises triglycerides levels, a type of fat in our blood. High HDL has a protective effect for cardiovascular diseases, but high amounts of triglycerides have the opposite effect. If you only drink wine occasionally as a treat, however, you can have relatively high HDL and an optimal ratio of total cholesterol to HDL.

4. Too many sweets: Sugar can be converted to triglycerides if it is not burned out as calories.

5. Imbalanced hormones: In a paper published in Human Reproduction 2009, women with polycyst ovarian syndrome, who do not ovulate regularly, tend to have high cholesterol with low HDL. This study suggests the role of hormones in regulating cholesterol and may explain one reason why women often develop high cholesterol after menopause.

Side effects of Statin drugs (including Lipitor and Zocor):

The recent withdrawal of Cerivastatin from U.S. markets has brought more attention to the side effects of Statin drugs. These include:

1. Liver damage: Did you know that your liver function can appear normal on lab tests even if liver damage has already occurred? Taking a Statin drug hurts your liver regardless of whether your liver function tests come back normal.

2. Muscle damage: Even if your blood serum creatine kinase (an important enzyme in muscle tissue) level is normal, you may still have muscle damage. In a clinical trial on Statin-associated muscle pain conducted by Dr. Paul Philips et al. in California, researchers stopped patients' Statin drug use for two weeks, then gave them Statin for another two weeks, and finally stopped it again. One participant had developed muscle aches and decreased exercise tolerance during 4 years of therapy with the Statin drug, Simvastatin. She found it difficult to ascend one flight of stairs without resting to relieve her leg ache. Two weeks after stopping the medication during the clinical trial, the symptoms were gone. Her muscle aches and hip weakness, however, recurred within 48 hours of reinitiating the Statin drug. Again, the patient's symptoms improved 3 months after discontinuing Statin therapy the second time. Muscle pain correlated directly with the use of Statin drugs.

3. Memory loss due to brain cell damage: Cholesterol is very important for protecting brain cells.

4. Neuropathy: If the nerves lose their protection due to low cholesterol levels, they will become inflamed and more vulnerable to infection.

5. ALS: When the nerves lose their protection, they also become more vulnerable to autoantibody attacks. Since we all have a certain amount of autoantibodies circulating in our blood, why do some people develop autoimmune diseases, whereas others do not? Two factors can contribute to the development of the diseases: one is how much auto antibodies a person has; the other is how healthy the protection layer of the nerves is. If an unhealthy diet already makes your immune function out of balance for a long time, the amount of autoantibody reaches certain level, and the long term use of the statin drug rips off the protection layer of the nerves, a person tends to develop this disease.

6. Depression, road rage, and extraordinary hostility: If the nerves cannot communicate properly, our mood will be out of whack.

7. Migraines: If there is not enough cholesterol to protect blood vessel walls, fluids may leak out of them, and they may become very sensitive to temperature and other environmental changes. The abnormal constriction or dilation of blood vessels causes migraines.

For more information, please check www.spacedoc.net. In this website, Dr. Duane Graveline, a former NASA astronaut, former USAF flight surgeon, and retired family doctor, indicates that reduced cholesterol production can also lead to decreased amounts of coenzyme Q10, a chemical very important to our heart health. Furthermore, Dr. Uffe Ravnskov has noted through scientific papers that although in general people have been taking in less saturated fat in the past 20 years, more and more people are developing Type II diabetes and having strokes.

Why do symptoms show up only after many years of taking Statin drugs?

Many patients say that they have been taking Statin drugs previously for many years without any problems. Although the damage had been taking place, they did not notice because the human body has a tremendous ability to compensate. Only when we reach the limit of compensation do the symptoms show.

Why do women have more side effects than men when they take Statin drugs?

Unlike men, women (especially menopausal or premenopausal women) can have instant side effects from Statin drugs, such as difficulty breathing and talking, and palpitations. Perhaps this occurs because cholesterol is the main precursor of progesterone, estrogen, and cortisol. Women tend to have a lowered level of cortisol after childbirth due to adrenal fatigue. If their cortisol and progesterone levels drop slightly because a Statin drug suppresses their cholesterol, their blood pressure, blood sugar, stress-coping ability, and mental status can change dramatically. Furthermore, most data regarding Lipitor come from male volunteers. Simply not enough data exist to show how Statin drugs influence women.

At my practice, many women come to me complaining of shoulder and hip pain, stroke-like symptoms, palpitations, and difficulty breathing. One patient tried several different Statin drugs, each time with the same result: she always ended up in the emergency room with slurred speech, palpitations, dizziness, and weakness. In addition, the muscle pain triggered by Statin drugs usually responds neither to physical therapy nor massage but to acupuncture. As long as these women took Statin drugs, I recommended they continue acupuncture.

How can you lower your cholesterol by changing your diet?

Cut down your intake of sweets such as cake, chocolate, and refined carbohydrates because simple sugars increases your triglycerides levels.

Reduce your alcohol intake to one or two glasses per week to get an optimized HDL level while maintaining a normal total cholesterol level. Other benefits of drinking less include better sleep and improved memory by protecting your nerves from alcohol damage.

Add flax seed and oats to your soup every day. Viscous fibers from those foods can increase the removal of cholesterol.

Eat a lot of vegetables to help discharge extra self-produced cholesterol from your body.

Oatmeal contains a natural ingredient called β-glucan that lowers our cholesterol level. If you eat oatmeal with the lowest amount of sugar for breakfast for 6 months, you may be able to lower your cholesterol level naturally. However, most types of oatmeal contain as much as 10 teaspoons of sugar in one serving.

Nutrium is a food supplement that has two times as much β-glucan as oatmeal to block the production of cholesterol before it reaches your blood stream. Please remember that your own body produces the majority of your cholesterol.

Red rice yeast from traditional Chinese medicine works in the same way as Statin drugs but has much weaker effect. You can take red yeast rice to lower your cholesterol level if changing your life style alone cannot bring your cholesterol level to the optimal level.

Take the lowest possible effective dosage of the medication if your lifestyle changes only work to a certain degree. According to Dr. Duane Graveline, in 1960, the average dose of Statin drugs was 15 mg/day but increased to 22 mg/day by 2003.

Clinical Case Study for High Cholesterol and Statin Drugs:

Mr. Lin, a graduate of Harvard Business School, worked in the financial industry. As a businessman, he had to eat at restaurants many times a week. He also loved to drink wine every evening. Although he was physically fit from his former training as a gymnast, at the age of forty-five, his cholesterol started climbing. His physician automatically prescribed Lipitor, and he had been taking that for more than five years before coming to see me.

At his wife's urging, he received acupuncture for the back muscle spasm at the T11 and T12 level he developed when lifting something during a ski trip. The pain was so severe that he could hardly move around, but if he took painkillers, he would be drowsy and unable to function well at work, which requires high mental acuity.

While treating his back muscle spasm, I found out that he had migraines quite often. In addition, his sleep was often interrupted: he would wake up in the middle of the night, spend an hour reading, and usually be unable to fall back asleep. Without sufficient sleep, he craved sweets to make him feel calm because sleep deprivation increased his cortisol level while depleting his feel-good hormones, such as serotonin and endorphin. He also developed tendonitis in his right elbow even though he does not play tennis or golf very often. His ski trips in the winter puts a lot of pressure on his right knee on which he had already received several surgeries. His migraines and knee and elbow pain all indicated that he had some kind of inflammation.

Degeneration of the joints usually starts at the age of sixty to sixty five, so something was causing them to degenerate abnormally early. First, I recommended several articles to him about how Lipitor inhibits the production of cholesterol, thereby causing dysfunction of cell membranes and blood vessel walls. He was very surprised to learn that, without the right level of cholesterol, cell membranes can leak fluids and easily develop inflammation in our muscles, nerves, and blood vessels. Then, I suggested that he cut down his wine intake. He was so determined to fix his problems that he completely stopped drinking alcohol within 3 months of his first acupuncture treatment.

Furthermore, I advised that he reduce his intake of simple sugars, which was difficult because his workplace always had candies and cookies available. Therefore, it was crucial that he got rid of all the sweets from his house so that he would not eat even more sugar when he came home, especially after dinner when his metabolism and physical activity is low. At night, these simple sugars are quickly converted into fat if our bodies do not burn them. Instead, if he rewarded himself with sweets only once every week and only after exercising, he could consume simple sugars without sacrificing his health.

Giving up simple sugar is a slow process because it is a strong habit. Sugar brings us instant satisfaction. This satisfaction is short-lived, but the damage it does to our blood vessels and nerve cells is irreversible. We need to find something else to bring us happiness. With an acupuncture treatment once a week, for example, our body can produce more of its own feel-good chemicals: the hormones dopamine, endorphin and serotonin.

After a year of acupuncture, Mr. Lin dramatically changed his eating habits. When he went out for business dinners in the evening, he would choose salad with vinegar dressing, brown rice and fruit for dessert. As for alcohol, he would sip a little bit at business dinners once or twice a week. In this way, he enjoyed his wine while keeping his mind clear and in control. Thankfully, in America, you do not need to drink heavily to do business. In China, on the other hand, in order to be someone's business partner, you have to empty your glass every time someone cheers. In the end, everyone gets drunk and has permanent liver damage. My uncle died in his early 30s from severe GI bleeding due to liver cirrhosis because he had been drinking this way for 10 years.

Three months after starting acupuncture and implementing dietary changes, Mr. Lin stopped taking Lipitor and changed to red yeast supplements, one capsule per day. His cholesterol level became normal and his HDL optimal. His inflammation was reduced with decreased intake of alcohol and sugar, and his elbow, knee, and back pains were controlled by acupuncture treatments once a week.

Like Lipitor, red yeast supplement inhibits the function of certain enzymes to reduce our body's production of cholesterol. The only difference is that red yeast is a traditional Chinese herb, a natural product used for thousands of years to treat digestive problems. Even so, if we take red yeast for too long in large doses, we can potentially have insufficient cholesterol in our bodies. Therefore, although the red yeast is a natural herb, it should still be used at the lowest effective dosage.

Mr. Lin made numerous lifestyle adjustments but I recently found out that he was having ice cream every night during the summer, which can potentially increase his total cholesterol level. To warn him of the dangers of this habit, I told him a story about two marathon runners I knew who ate ice cream daily for many years. One day, their physicians found out that their coronary arteries were blocked more than 80%, and they immediately underwent quadruple bypass surgeries. After surgery, they did not change their diets but started taking Lipitor instead. Five years later, one patient developed ALS and the other strange immune problems. He had no γ-globulin in his body and needed a $10,000 infusion of γ-globulin every other month. Although both of them now try to eat healthily, the damage caused by the sugar and saturated fat in ice cream has become permanent, so their symptoms may improve but will never go away.

Is high cholesterol a disease? Why do so many Centenarians have High Cholesterol but suffer no Strokes?

Dr. John Lee and other physicians say that high cholesterol itself is not the main reason for the blockage of blood vessels. It is inflammation, which changes the structure of the inner layer of blood vessels that causes cholesterol to accumulate underneath, forming plaques. Most people who live up to 90 years old without severe medical conditions eat a high fiber diet, walk every day, and do not have sweets regularly. Therefore, although many of these people do have high cholesterol, it does not result in a stroke. Back in the 1970's, my paternal grandfather had three brothers who lived in the countryside. They hardly ever ate any sweets or meat and all lived into their nineties in good health. My grandfather, on the other hand, who was much better off financially, started eating sweets every day after turning 70, developed pancreatic cancer several years later, and died at age 82 in severe pain, because inflammation not only causes strokes but also cancer.

Why do so many women develop stroke in their forties or fifties?

More and more women are taking artificial hormones to help regulate their periods or menopause symptoms. Dr. Caroline Dean cites many studies linking the birth control pill and stroke in women. The mechanism for this correlation may be associated with altered cholesterol levels, inflamed blood vessels, and imbalanced immune function.

Chinese Herbal Formula to optimize cholesterol level:

1. Spleen deficiency with accumulating phlegm:

Symptoms: High cholesterol, overweight, fatigue, sleep more than eight hours a night, irregular periods, overgrowing facial and leg hair, foggy head, and cysts in various areas.

Tongue: puffy with a greasy white or yellow coating. Pulse: soggy.

Formula: Gua Lou 15g, Sheng Shan Zha 15g, Ban Xia 12g, Chen Pi 6g, Yuan Zhi 12g, Jiao Shan Zha 15g, Zhi Shi 12g, Yin Chen 30g, Sheng Mai Ya 15g.

2. Liver and kidney Yin deficiency with deficient heat:

Symptoms: Normal weight, night sweats, bottoms of the feet and palms feel hot, irritability, thirsty all the time.

Formula: Zhi Shou Wu 30g, Huang Jing 10g, Jue Ming Zi 30g, Sheng Yi Yi Ren 30g, Yin Chen 24g, Ze Xie 24g, Sheng Shan Zha 18g, Chai Hu 12g, Yu Jin 12g, Jiu Da Huang 6g.

Acupuncture points to normalize your metabolism and to prevent food from being converted into fat:

SP15 (Da Heng): 4 cun lateral to belly button.

CV9: On the anterior median line of the upper abdomen, 1.0 cun above the belly button.

TW6: On the dorsal aspect of the forearm, 3 cun above the transverse crease of the wrist between the ulna and radius.

ST40: 8 cun superior to the external malleolus, two finger-breadth from the anterior crest of the tibia.

Chapter Five

Irritable Bowel

Syndrome (IBS)

I f you read the information regarding IBS, you will find the following: "Although there is no cure for IBS there are treatments that attempt to relieve symptoms, including dietary adjustments, medication and psychological interventions. Patient education and a good doctor-patient relationship are also important. The exact cause of IBS is unknown. The most common theory is that IBS is a disorder of the interaction between the brain and the gastrointestinal tract, although there may also be abnormalities in the gut flora or the immune system. What I do and what all practitioners of Traditional Chinese Medicine do is to teach you self-healing techniques most would give up hope of a cure, but don't; read on and be cured.

Interestingly, IBS and its treatment provide a good example of the differences in treatment and philosophy between western medicine and Traditional Chinese Medicine. There is a clue for this inconvenient condition, which reminds us how important our regular bowel movement is. We establish enough of a relationship with our patients so we understand not only their symptoms, but what about THEM and their life is causing their ailment.

Since this ailment can be described as an "interaction" of systems, it requires an understanding of how the systems relate and what about that relationship can effect improvement in the condition. A patient may not have one root cause that can be treated with a pill. She may need to change the way she eats, when to eat, what to eat, how much to eat. She may need to make a lifestyle change by getting more sleep, or deal with stress by working fewer hours or doing something a bit different. The doctor needs to spend the time to understand the components of the problem, not just give the diagnose of this disease. Traditional Chinese Medicine is used to treat not only the symptoms, but also the root cause, such as the imbalance of each organ or system. Herbs or acupuncture may be used as well as lifestyle changes but I consider the way a person leads his/her life as the chief suspect contributor to the problem, especially for a sickness such as IBS.

There is much research about the mechanism and causes of IBS in Pubmed, the official site for the clinical and basic scientific researches. So let me get a little technical on you for a bit. The symptoms of IBS are diarrhea, or diarrhea alternates with constipation, bloating, gas, indigestion, unpleasant smell in the mouth, abdominal cramping relieved after a bowel movement.

The mechanism for how this works is an imbalance of chemicals in the digestive system along with nervous system abnormalities causing hypersensitivity and a resultant abnormal movement of the intestines. Bowel movements are controlled by the central nervous system and the intestinal nervous system, called the enteric nervous system, located underneath the mucous membrane and smooth muscles. Sympathetic nerves inhibit intestinal motility and secretion and cause contraction of the sphincters and blood vessels. Thus if you are always on the run and you never relax, your digestive system will not get enough blood circulation, your enzyme production will become inhibited and intestinal movement becomes abnormal with constipation and indigestion. On the other hand, the parasympathetic nervous system (the relaxing part of the nervous system) makes your body relax and digest. At night, the parasympathetic nervous system is dominant. You go to bed, relax and digest food thoroughly. When you lie down, your stomach makes noise due to increased regular movement to digest food. Two chemicals can influence bowel movement: acetylcholine and norepinephrine. Acetylcholine enhances the intestinal movement while norepinephine inhibits it. The balance of these two chemicals and other chemicals facilitates regular bowel movement.

IBS affects about 12% of the population in the United States and is increasing at a 2% rate each year. So why has IBS become so common in the United States?

1. Changed sleep patterns: our digestive system needs to repair every night. Growth hormone secretion increases after 8 PM and reaches the highest level between 2 AM to 4 AM during your deep sleep. If you go to bed as late as 2 AM, the majority of your deep sleep time will be shifted and your body will not produce enough growth hormone causing your intestinal membrane to miss its repair window which would have allowed the body to recover from heavy-duty digestion during the day. Before Thomas Edison invented the light bulb, people went to bed once it turned dark and the average sleep time for an American was 8 to 9 hours.

2. Having a big meal after 7 PM causes indigestion, the undigested food becomes a toxin leading to intestinal membrane inflammation.

3. Cigarettes inflame the intestinal membrane. The excuse that some people used to continue smoking was its effect on weight. Part of that is true, an inflamed intestinal wall does not digest food well and therefore the body does not process that food. But if they eat cookies instead, they could still be overweight, because junk food does not need a healthy intestine to digest.

4. Alcohol can cause inflammation in the digestive and nervous systems, leading to irregular bowel movement. There are many nerves embedded underneath the intestinal membrane. If they are inflamed, they can become very sensitive to environmental and food stimulation. Many alcoholics cannot eat vegetables, which need a highly complex digestion process; they get bloating very easily.

5. Caffeine can stimulate an irritable bowel. After you drink coffee, you may not get symptoms right away; it does overly sensitize your digestive system. That is why some people use coffee to fix their constipation.

6. Tea can slow down your bowel movement. If you drink too much coffee in the morning, then drink very strong tea in the afternoon; you really confuse your digestive system.

7. Eating sweets can lead to inflammation. When you eat sweets, you feel happy at that moment. This happiness only lasts for a couple of hours, and then you need another fix. You will not be able to feel the effects of the inflammation until your body cannot compensate any more.

8. Medications: pain killers, high blood pressure medication, sleeping pills and anti-depressives can cause constipation, then you have to use laxatives, which make your intestines contract intensely.

Alternating between constipation and diarrhea makes your bowel movement very irregular.

10. Too much spicy food: In Chinese medicine, spicy food produces internal heat, causing inflammation. With all the stress we have, almost everybody has blocked energy somewhere, which is linked with internal heat. That is why we should not eat too much spicy food to aggravate this condition. In modern society, city living increases our stress; historically humans have not had as much stress as today, therefore energy was not blocked and our bodies did not produce excessive heat, so eating spicy foods could help an undernourished body produce more heat.

11. Too many raw vegetables: most raw vegetables cannot be digested well in our stomach and intestines even though many people claim that the raw ones contain more nutrients. If your body cannot break down the raw fibers, they become harmful to your intestinal membrane and stimulate your bowl movement.

12. Ice cold water can also cause indigestion because it makes the digestive enzymes work less efficiently, especially when you eat spicy or greasy food.

13. Over thinking can shut down the blood flow to your stomach and intestines and cause irregular bowel movement and indigestion.

14. Lack of fiber: People who develop IBS are afraid of eating fiber, thinking it will stimulate their bowel movement. Without the fiber to increase intestinal movement, they develop constipation. Then they use a laxative, which often can lead to diarrhea.

15. Too much stress: Stress can be caused by too much of anything: information, food, too much thinking, too much noise without the body and mind processing it. Stress increases cortisol and adrenaline causing a dysfunction of the digestive system.

The simple way to resolve your IBS:

Drink warm water a half hour before your meal, no ice-cold water during the meal, especially when you are eating greasy or spicy food.

Eat cooked vegetables, especially cauliflower, broccoli, or celery; you can steam or stir-fried them in order to deal with diarrhea. Once your symptoms are gone, try a small amount of raw salad every other day and adjust to find out the right amount you can tolerate.

Making this porridge to strengthen your digestive function:

Add a half-gallon of water, 30g of Chinese Yams, 30g of Yi Yi Ren (Semen coicis), a half cup of brown rice in the crock-pot and cook over night. Have a bowl of this porridge every morning.

Add fresh ginger in your soup to help your digestion. Dried sugary ginger is not good.

Raw Cucumbers are very effective to improve digestion. You can also add vinegar in your cucumber salad.

Go to bed around 11PM and get up around 6 AM. This will help regulate your hormone and nervous system in order to optimize your digestive function.

Avoid spicy food, raw garlic and onion when your diarrhea flares up. Once you are healed, you can introduce them little by little. Lightly cooked garlic and onion are better for digestion.

Do not eat cold meat, large amount of nuts or dairy products if you have IBS symptoms. The intestines are in a very sensitive state, any food which is hard to digest can trigger diarrhea.

Peel fruit before you eat it, the skin has a lot of fiber, which may cause bloating and diarrhea if you have IBS.

Try to have dinner before 6 PM, eating late itself can cause indigestion. If you do not have time to cook dinner, you can have a whole wheat sandwich and later eat very light dinner.

Case Study:

When I first met Susan, she was a jovial 60 year old, woman. Nothing seems to bother her. She loved to cook and eat. She enjoyed friends, and was easy to talk to. Her difficult health problems did not seem to bother her. In retrospect, I'm sure she had all the life stresses and difficult things to deal with that we all do. No one escapes a bit of that. But Susan never showed that side of herself in all the time I saw her. If things were not going her way during a particular day, she would still come to my office with a happy face. It was not that she was insensitive; I believe she felt things deeply. She just kept all of that to herself.

When many of us think of Chinese Medicine we think of herbs and acupuncture. However, much of how I treat a person's ailment, does not depend on these tools. I am interested in what life situation or habits influence the problem. And I allow the patient to play a bit part in their own healing by slightly changing what they do every day. They can change in a small way what they eat or drink. They can pay attention to how much sleep they get and how they get ready for sleep. Are they taking on too much at work leading to excessive stress or lack of sleep? Are there environmental problems in their house or workplace that should be avoided? I try to see their whole life in my mind and how it affects their problems.

Susan ate ice cream every day and put sugar and cream into her coffee. She slept well and had had good digestion until she reached 40 years of age. Due to a hormone imbalance after menopause, she developed *in situ* cancer in her vaginal area in 1975. In 1980, her gallbladder was removed because of an infection. In 1989 she had two herniated discs, one was ruptured. She had a back operation right away. In 1999, she had a heart attack resulting in angio-plastic surgery. She subsequently had a series of other surgeries to mend her heart problems. No one told her that she should stop eating ice cream or other sweets every day. She was still overweight and went out to eat twice a week. She did not know that essentially ice cream equals sugar plus fat and could re-block her coronary arteries far faster that other types of foods.

When she came to me in May of 2009, she had been plagued with chronic diarrhea for many years. She was diagnosed with celiac condition initially, meaning her intestinal membranes were all inflamed and she could not digest a kind of protein in flour called gluten. Her immune function was out of balance. She had to eat gluten free food, which was very expensive. She was allergic to soy and sugar substitutes. If she ate a high salt diet, her knee and ankles became swollen. She could not sleep well, and kept gaining weight even with diarrhea as much as eight times a day. The undigested food became stored as fat tissue instead of providing her body heat and vital energy. She loved to pick up her friends from the airport, but with all her illnesses, she had been worried about getting to a restroom in time. After all the medication and surgeries, she went to a support group. There it was suggested she try acupuncture. Her friend called me and set up an appointment for her.

At her intake visit, I collected all of her dieting information and suggested that she eliminate chocolates and other simple sugars. My theory was that those sweets do not need enzymes to be digested. So you never feel full without fiber, protein and oil in your stomach. The sweets stimulate your brain to produce dopamine just like alcohol, you feel happy at the time. The worst thing is that you cannot see the damage until the sweets inflame the majority of your blood vessels and nerves. That is why even though she ate quite healthy foods overall , and took her medication faithfully, she still could not get rid of her IBS. Her passions for sweets including ice cream made her cholesterol go up and caused inflammation of her coronary artery and intestinal membranes. That was why she developed a heart attack and celiac disease in her early forties. Lipitor artificially lowered her cholesterol. While she continued her unhealthy sweets eating, the systematic inflammation continued even as her blood work showed normal cholesterol levels. The diarrhea medication controlled the symptoms initially, but the inflammation got worse and worse, and eventually the medication could not help any more. She had a long list of food, which went right through her intestines: coffee, tea, cream, cereals, wheat, rye, oats, and alcohol. Even certain brands of conditioner caused her scalp sores. She felt bloated around her middle and had no energy all the time. However, she could eat steamed or toasted vegetables, fruit, well cooked meat and dairy. Her body could not digest the gluten very well.

Potatoes do not have long fibers, so it can be absorbed quickly. Right after you eat potatoes, your blood sugar goes up above the normal level, causing inflammation in your nerves and blood vessels, encouraging infection and cancer growth. Her sudden energy drop was also associated with her sharp fluctuations of blood sugar. The systematic chronic inflammation has been verified to stimulate cancer cell growth, remember fast growing cells need sugar to feed them.

The next step was analyzing her three meals. She started her morning with banana and yogurt, which has a lot of sugar. Then she ate an apple with peanut butter, which also has some sugar. She knew that her coffee caused diarrhea, but she continued to drink it. So I recommended that she stop drinking coffee. She later found that certain brands of coffee were OK if she only had one cup without sugar substitute. My suggestion was to choose no sugar yogurt and eat an apple without peanut butter.

Looking back on her treatments:

After only two treatments, she did not get diarrhea for four days. The following week, she went to an expensive restaurant with her friend, and she had a spinach salad for dinner, and the next morning her diarrhea returned. So I told her not to eat raw vegetables until she was diarrhea free for a while. She followed my advice. After the fourth treatment, she did not have diarrhea for a week.

She was thrilled about the changes in her health; in the mean time her swollen knees, ankles and shoulder pain were improving with lowered salt intake. Then she started eating hot dogs, some onions, and peppers in a party, the next morning she had diarrhea. I suggest she eat cooked peppers and onions to see if she develops diarrhea. Later I found out she still eats ice cream every day to make her happy. Her husband developed Parkinson's disease in his fifties; He had been taking medication to control his tremor. Without changing his diet, his brain cells continued to be damaged by sweets. Now the brain cells are not responding to the medication. He can hardly walk without his wife's help. His physician decided to implant a stimulator in his brain and constant stimulation may make his brain cells respond to the medication again, so that he can walk with help.

Susan had to take her husband in and out of the hospital numerous times to get different tests. She was stressed out, that is why she ate so much ice cream to make her happy. I told her that if you want your husband to get better, you have to set a good example and stop eating sweets every day. Otherwise Susan may develop another heart attack in the near future and her husband may not even walk with the implanted device in his brain. At that point, she stopped eating ice cream, other sweets, and coffee with cream. Her diarrhea stopped for 10 days. After her diarrhea went away for more than two weeks, she went out to eat at her regular restaurant; she even ate scallops with certain natural spices. She had no diarrhea afterward.

Her snack now is crackers with fruit and orange juice, not ice cream or chocolate. The next step was getting rid of all the hidden sugar to stop the systematic inflammation in her body. Instead of drinking orange juice, she has an orange regularly. She only had ice cream occasionally. After six treatments with all the dieting changes, she did not have diarrhea for 17 days. She also could eat home cooked pork, chicken, fish, cooked onions and different kinds of steamed vegetables, all without diarrhea. Her secret for eating meat without diarrhea was to remove all the fat on the meat. Considering her gallbladder was removed, it was quite amazing that she could still eat different kinds of meat and digest them properly. At that point, she only drank a certain brand of coffee, which she could tolerate, one cup twice a week, but she did stop putting cream and sugar into her coffee and she stopped eating pears, which very often caused bloating.

Due to being overweight and having inflamed blood vessels for many years, her varicose veins were very pronounced on her left inner thigh. There was no pain with these varicose veins, but she did not like how they looked. We started working on this problem. Because the varicose veins are right on the spleen channels, we could enhance spleen function and reduce varicose veins at the same time. Due to long time systematic inflammation, the pre-cancer changes came back, the gynecologist used acid to remove the pre-cancer tissue in her vaginal area, and the pain was so bad that she had to put oil into her vagina to reduce the burning pain while she was taking a bath. The oil made the bathtub so slippery that she fell into her bath tab and injured her left shoulder. But she was a very happy person despite all of these problems. With three additional acupuncture treatments, her big bruises and pain in her shoulder went away within a week. She was able to pick up her friends at the airport again. During her visit to Boston, she had a cup of ice coffee, she had diarrhea right after she finished her coffee. So she realized she had to be careful, even now.

Now she could go out to eat at a restaurant once a week. She had more energy and less bloating. She could enjoy a little bit of spicy food. Furthermore, her vaginal discomfort was gone after she changed her diet. Diarrhea flared up when she took antibiotics for her finger infection for 10 days. During that period of time, she tried to eat homemade food all the time. She was able to stop her diarrhea right after she stopped taking antibiotics.

At the end of 2009, Susan went on a cruise for three weeks; she had a few episodes of diarrhea due to her changed diet. But once she came back home, she had regular bowel movements. This meant that her intestinal inflammation had been dramatically improved, due to her healthy diet. Her body had quickly recovered from an unhealthy diet.

Chinese Herbal Formula:

1. Internal heat blocked in the intestines: smelly stool, constipation alternates with diarrhea, strong appetite, and increased bowl movement after eating greasy food. Tongue: bright red with yellow thick coating in the middle and back, pulse: slippery.

Herbal formula: Huang Bai 12g, Dang Gui 9g, Yi Yi ren 30g, Chi Shao 15g, Bai Zhu 15g, Fu Ling 15g, Huang Lian 6g, Di Yu 15g.

2. Liver Qi Stagnation: diarrhea gets worse with increased stress, irritability, mood swing, abdominal cramping, and pain gets relieved after bowel movement, mucous in the stool. Tongue: red, coating is white greasy or yellow greasy.

Herbal formula: Chai Hu 6g, Zhi Shi 9g, Bai shao 15g, Xiang Fu 6g, Wu Mei 6g, Zhi Gan Cao 3g, Chuan Lian Zi 6g, Fang Feng 10g, Bai Zhu 15g.

3. Spleen Qi deficiency: abdominal pain with bloating and gas, mucous in the stool, reduced appetite, sleep a lot, foggy head, pale complex, fatigue, no energy to talk. Tongue: pale, thin white coating. Pulse: thin, weak.

Herbal formula: Dang Shen 15g, Xian He Cao 15g, Bai Ji Li 10g, Chen Pi 10g, Di Yu 12g, Fu Ling 10g, Sha Ren 6g. Shan Zha 15g, Xi Yang Shen 6g, Lian Zi 15g, Shan Yao 30g.

4. Kidney qi deficiency: diarrhea more than 3 times a day especially early in the morning, abdominal aches with rumbling sound, pain gets better with heating pad and light pressure, urgent and frequent bowel movement, weight loss, fatigue, low back pain, reduced sexual drive, aversion to cold, joint pain. Tongue: pale with thin white coating, Pulse: deep thin.

Herbal formula: Huang Qi 30g, Wu Zei Gu 30g, Tu Si Zi 30g, Chao Bai Zhu 20g, Mu Xiang 12g, Chi Shi Zhi 24g, Shan Yao 30g, Chao Mai Ya 20g, Bu Gu Zhi 15g.

Acupuncture and IBS:

Scientific evidence:

The newest research in World J. Gastroenterol, 2009 indicated that Electrical acupuncture on ST25 (two inches next to belly button) and ST37 (6 inches below knee eye and one finger breath from the ridge of the tibia bone) can desensitize the nerves of intestine, increase the pain threshold by reducing the chemicals associated with pain sensation, and reduce the number of mast cells in colons, which release histamine and other inflammatory chemicals, causing cramp and diarrhea in rat IBS model.

The researchers at the Columbia University School of Nursing conducted studies on humans with IBS with acupuncture and moxa in a preliminary, randomized, sham/placebo-controlled trial. Twenty-nine men and women with IBS were randomized to either individualized Acu/Moxa (treatment group) or sham/placebo (control group). All subjects were assessed by a diagnostic acupuncturist for a traditional Chinese Medicine evaluation and individualized point prescription. Only those subjects assigned to the experimental group received the individually prescribed treatment. The diagnostic acupuncturist did not administer treatments and was blind to treatment assignments. All subjects kept a symptom diary for the duration of the study, enabling measurement of symptom frequency, severity, and improvement.

After 4 weeks of twice-weekly Acu/Moxa treatment, average daily abdominal pain/discomfort improved whereas the control group showed minimal reduction. This between-group difference adjusted for baseline difference was statistically significant. The findings indicate that Acu/Moxa treatment shows promise symptom management by balancing the nervous system and chemicals for IBS patients.

Then why didn't everybody get better by acupuncture treatment?

In the first rat study, acupuncture was applied daily for 7 days. The second human study gave the treatment twice a week for four weeks. A sufficient treatment number could have produced more satisfactory results. Also the personal dieting changes were also the key factor. If after an acupuncture treatment, the patients still eat very greasy, spicy food or too much dairy products, the inflamed intestinal membranes never have a chance to recover.

Another interesting study was published in Complementary Therapies in Medicine, 2007 by Schneider A et al. This study explained the differences of acupuncture and placebo effect. Patients with IBS were randomly assigned to receive either acupuncture or sham acupuncture using the so-called "Streitberger needle". The effects on the autonomic nervous system were evaluated by measuring salivary cortisol and by cardiovascular responses on a tilt table before and after 10 acupuncture treatments. The researchers found that the quality of life of the IBS patients increased in both groups with no group differences. Salivary cortisol decreased in all groups. However, the decrease was more pronounced in the acupuncture group. Heart rate response decreased on a tilt table in the acupuncture group while it increased in the sham acupuncture group, indicating an increased parasympathetic (the relaxing part of the nervous system) tone in the acupuncture group. Improvement of pain was positively associated with increased parasympathetic tone in the acupuncture group, but not in the sham acupuncture group. The acupuncture does have specific physiological effects compared to the unspecific improvement of quality of life in both real and sham acupuncture groups. Thus, different mechanisms seem to be involved in placebo and real-acupuncture driven improvements.

Then how can different acupuncture points are used to treat different symptoms of IBS? Dr. Takahashi T in Duke University medical school answered this question. He suggested that stimulating ST36 can enhance the intestinal motility, so it relives indigestion, acid reflex and can be a good treatment for constipation dominant IBS. While stimulating CV12 relaxes the stomach and intestinal smooth muscles, it can be used to treat diarrhea of IBS.

Effective Acupuncture points for IBS:

CV7 (Yin Jiao): On the anterior median line of the lower abdomen, 1.0 cun below the belly button.

CV9 (Shui Fen): On the anterior median line of the upper abdomen, 1.0 cun above the belly button.

Diarrhea point 1 (extra points): 1 inch next to belly button.

ST37 (Shang Ju Xu): On the anterior aspect of the lower leg, 6 cun below internal knee eye, one finger-breadth (middle finger) from the anterior crest of the tibia.

IBS with constipation, diarrhea, abdominal pain, flank pain, and acid reflex:

Diarrhea points 2 (extra point): half inch below belly button

CV15 (Jiu Wei): On the anterior median line of the upper abdomen, 1.0 cun below the xiphisternal synchondroses, especially with symptoms of heart burn and stomach ache.

ST36 (Zu San Li): On the anterior aspect of the lower leg, 3 cun below internal knee eye, one finger-breadth (middle finger) from the anterior crest of the tibia.

CV12 (Zhong Wuan): On the anterior median line of the upper abdomen, 4.0 cun above the umbilicus.

ST25 (Tian Shu): 2 cun lateral to the belly button.

Liv13 (Zhang Men): On the lateral side of the abdomen, below the free end of the 11th floating rib.

If diarrhea alternates with constipation:

TW7: 3 cun above the transverse crease of the wrist between the ulna and radius.

If patient has frequent panic attack:

HT6: on the radial side of the tendon m. flexor carpi ulnaris, 0.5 cun above the transverse crease of the wrist.

Diarrhea with low back pain and low sexual drive:

Kid16 (Huang Shu): 0.5 cun next to belly button, needles point toward the center of belly button, insert needles 1.2 inches.

Moxa the area 1.5 inch below external malleolus twice a day for 15 to 30 min. alternating between left and right.

Chapter Six

Depression and Anxiety

What is depression really? Some say that depression is an illness involving the mind and the body and that because it affects how one feels, thinks, and behaves, depression can lead to a variety of emotional and physical problems such as sadness, irritability or frustration, reduced sexual drive, insomnia or excessive sleeping, changes in appetite, agitation or restlessness, slowed thinking, indecisiveness, distractibility, fatigue, and loss of energy.

Depression affects 26.2 % of all Americans, which means that when you board a bus to work in the morning, one in every four passengers is clinically depressed. It is a hidden illness that often goes undiagnosed and untreated because we can easily blame its symptoms on something else. Thus, we spend a lifetime convincing ourselves that when we say day after day, "I am so tired; I don't feel like going out. I'm not hungry, sexually motivated, or interested enough to participate," it is just a defect in our personality.

Depression changes people close to us. Loved ones can feel a loss of emotional connection with someone who is depressed. Friends at work may have to put in extra hours to make up for the loss of productivity when their co-workers' depression interferes with their job.

Western medicine has created drugs, which successfully treat many types of depression and anxiety. Because these drugs are so powerful, however, suddenly starting, stopping, or changing dosage can lead to unpredictable outcomes. Children and young adults, especially, may react to these medications in ways not predicted by FDA trials. On the other hand, Chinese medicine, which uses the body and mind's own mechanisms to combat depression, may be a safer first approach to less severe cases since innate systems are tweaked rather than radically altered.

The following chapter explores depression chiefly as an imbalance of hormones such as, GABA, dopamine, epinephrine, norepinephrine, and progesterone.

What causes depression?

Irregular sleep: Cortisol levels should go up in the morning while melatonin goes down. If your melatonin level is high at the wrong time, however, you may feel groggy and depressed. For example, if you take a long nap in the middle of the day, you may wake up feeling tired and unhappy for the next two hours. Moreover, this nap may further offset your sleep rhythm because when bedtime comes, you are still not sleepy.

Unhealthy diet: If your body does not have enough raw materials to produce what I call the "feel good hormones," serotonin, progesterone, GABA, and dopamine, to relax your mind and body, you will not feel well no matter how rich or loved you are.

Alcohol: Alcohol can cause sudden increases of your dopamine level. When you are hung over the next morning, however, your body experiences a sudden drop in dopamine, and therefore you feel depressed. It's like having bipolar disorder: one moment you feel high due to a higher level of feel good hormones but the next moment the hormones are depleted so you just as suddenly become depressed.

Lack of exercise: Not exercising can lead to insufficient β-endorphin and serotonin production. Without exercise, there would not be sufficient blood flow to nourish your internal organs. When these organs do not function well, you have less feel good hormones.

Anti-acids: Anti-acids can cause a deficiency of vitamins and mal-absorption of proteins, leading to an abnormally functioning nervous system, which becomes supersensitive to the physical and mental stress. Therefore, you cannot relax and enjoy life. In my experience, I have noticed that people who already have problems with anxiety and depression tend to have more panic attacks after they take anti-acids for a period of the time.

Caffeine: Drinking too much caffeine stimulates your "fight or flight" system constantly, causing you to always rush around from one thing to another. When you attempt to multitask, you tend to become more anxious.

Indigestion: Even if you eat a healthy diet, if your stomach cannot digest it well, ultimately, you will not get enough nutrients to produce balanced levels of hormones. Instead, the undigested food can become toxic to your body.

Aging: When people become older, their digestive system also goes downhill. Thus, if they do not eat a very balanced diet, their bodies may not absorb the nutrients necessary to produce enough feel good hormones. Cakes, cookies, and ice cream can only make them happy for a short period of time. These junk foods not only impede their digestion but also deplete their supply of feel good hormones.

Stress: Stress makes people produce too much cortisol and adrenaline, the "fight or flight" hormones, causing a chemical imbalance and thus depression and anxiety.

Lack of sunshine: Daytime sunlight can reset the circadian cycle of melatonin, which influences our mood.

Adrenal fatigue: After exposure to long-term stress, the adrenal gland can no longer provide enough of the stress-coping hormones cortisol and progesterone so that the slightest environmental change can make you feel anxious and depressed. Trauma, such as car accidents, can trigger a sudden release of adrenaline and cortisol, depleting adrenal gland function and your reserve of relaxing hormones such as serotonin, GABA, progesterone, and dopamine.

How can you prevent or eliminate depression?

1. Avoid multitasking: Shut your cell phone off when driving or spending time with a family member. You will feel calmer if you do one thing after another. In the long run, by making fewer mistakes, you will save time and feel happier and more productive.

2. Optimize your sleep time: Serotonin levels fluctuate rhythmically on a circadian 24- hour cycle. Thus, if you go to bed and wake up at the wrong times, your normal chemical balance will be disturbed. Clinically, most depressed people tend to sleep very late at

night and rise very late in the morning. When they make an effort to go to bed early and get up with the sun, their depression decreases dramatically. Therefore, if you do not feel tired at bedtime, try doing yoga or meditation or reading a boring book in order to induce sleep at the right time. You can also practice Qigong or Taichi or simply stretch an hour before bed. In my experience, morning birds that get sufficient sleep during their prime sleeping hours are less likely to get depressed than night owls.

3. Sleep enough: Get enough sleep to rejuvenate your endocrine, nervous, and digestive functions so that your relaxing and stimulating hormones are in balance.

4. Reduce caffeine intake: Try to find the perfect amount of coffee that is just enough to wake you up in the morning but not so much to make you anxious. Never drink coffee in the evening because it will profoundly influence your nervous system and make you unhappy the next day.

5. Improve your digestion: Add apple cedar vinegar to your salad or put daikon or wheat bran into your soup. Do not skip meals or eat too late or too much. Avoid consuming too many sweets, which may slow down digestion. Eat one banana in the afternoon every day to provide your body with enough tryptophan, the precursor of serotonin.

106

You will sleep better because serotonin makes our sleep deep and sound.

6. Have regular sex: Sex improves the production of progesterone and testosterone, both of which help us stay happy and healthy.

7. Step outside: Get enough sunshine every day to boost your endorphin production and to reset your internal biological clock.

8. Sing: Singing enhances your lung capacity and improves the oxygen saturation of your internal organs. A 94-year-old MIT professor started singing only 3 days after 1/3 of his lung was removed due to tuberculosis. He recovered much faster than other patients who did not share his passion for singing.

9. Try something new: Join different social activities such as volunteering at a hospital and you will find how fulfilling your life is when you interact with others.

How can you improve your serotonin level naturally?

Nutrition:

Serotonin is sensitive to dietary intake. If you increase your consumption of tryptophan, the chemical from which serotonin is made; your body can produce more serotonin. Tryptophan can be found in a variety of foods such as turkey, bananas, milk, yogurt, eggs, meat, nuts, beans, fish, cheddar, and Gruyere and Swiss cheeses. Because this substance also acts as a mild sedative on the human body, it is no wonder that after a big Thanksgiving dinner, everybody feels so sleepy and hopefully happy.

Exercise:

As shown in an article published in Endocrinology 2007 by French physician, Dr. Z.S. Malek, enhanced voluntary locomotion during a 6-week period increased serotonin production level in normal rats without a concomitant increase in plasma cortisol levels. Because serotonin levels increase in the blood during exercise, mild depression may be relieved by moderate physical exercise.

Food Therapy:

Happy Porridge (for people with depression, indigestion, and low sexual drive): Put half gallon of water, ¼ cup of lotus seed, ¼ cup of walnuts, ½ cup of brown rice, and ¼ cup of black bean together in a slow cooker and let cook for six hours.

If you suffer from depression with insomnia, add 30g of Suan Zao Ren (Ziziphus) and 30g of Yi Yi Ren (Job's tears) to the Happy Porridge.

Clinical Case Study:

TL is a famous geophysicist who wrote 5 books and published more than 100 scientific papers. Born in a small town in northeastern China to parents who could neither read nor write, by talent and hard work alone, he was accepted into Beijing University, which, founded by Americans in the 1920's, was the most prestigious university in China. He was very athletic during high school and college, playing soccer and speed skating for the university team. After graduation, he started doing research for the Chinese Scientific Institute, working more than 12 hours a day for many years.

Generally, he ate very healthily, but he had two bad habits that may have contributed to his health condition later in life. One was that he ate too many sweets. Sixty years ago in the 1950s, each person in China was allotted only 1.3 pounds of white sugar every month. Professor TL would finish his ration in one sitting. In the past twenty years, after sugar became more available, he would usually eat cookies every evening before dinner and hardly any vegetables during the meal. The second contributor to his health condition was not drinking enough water.

When TL was young, he would periodically have migraines so severe that he would be forced to lie down and cover all the windows for a couple of hours. During those times, he would not talk to anybody.

He also had chronic low blood pressure his entire life, so he would have to take short naps every day after lunch in order to function efficiently in the afternoon. Nevertheless, his health was fair until he reached 60 years of age.

At 60, he started suffering from knee pain that got progressively worse and worse. Interestingly enough, his knees would not hurt at all during the daytime while he was active, but would only bother him at night. When he lied down, severe pain along with a cold sensation would permeate both knees and the tops of his ankles. He struggled with the pain and refused to take sleeping pills or painkillers, tossing and turning until around 2 AM, when he would fall into an exhausted sleep for 4 hours. With this kind of severe pain, one would expect that his X-rays would show major changes in the knees. Yet surprisingly, his knees exhibited only mild degeneration compared to most other people his age. Although his knee pain did not interfere with his daily physical activities, it prevented him from resting well because it would always come back whenever he sat or lied down. I discovered that rather than a structural problem, his knee pain was rooted in the dysfunction of his nervous system because the insertion of acupuncture needles would cause his knees to twitch intermittently.

I learned from his personal history that although he would eat five apples a day when he was young, in his early fifties, he stopped eating most kinds of fruits and vegetables because his teeth started falling out. His favorite foods became bread and cookies. Over the years, this diet led to a deficiency of vitamins and minerals, thus causing his nervous system to become overly sensitive and to greatly amplify even the slightest pain signal. Although he had been a brave man most of his life, fighting the Japanese who had invaded China and leading Chinese scientists to different countries, he had his first panic attack at the age of 65. While sitting on the subway to escort his granddaughter to a dance class, he suddenly felt so nauseous and dizzy that he got out of the subway as soon as possible, leaving his granddaughter to go to downtown Boston by herself. Gradually, he developed anxiety and depression.

TL's symptoms of depression first started when he returned to China to visit his colleagues and finish up his research after living in the U.S. for 3 years. His face would suddenly turn red, and he would have hot flashes for a few minutes. Every night, he would remember his mistakes from the past and, regretting those things; he would slap his face repeatedly. Instead of taking anti-depressants like the Chinese doctors prescribed, he came back to the U.S. upon his daughter's suggestion and continued teaching his grandchildren Chinese and math. After returning, his depression gradually got better and within a couple of months, his hot flushes also disappeared.

TL is not a happy person because he isolated himself after retirement. Although he used to lead a group of scientist, predicting earthquakes and traveling to many countries, when he stopped doing research, he refused to join any senior activities and gave up all his hobbies.

In this case, TL's pain, claustrophobia, insomnia, depression, and hot flashes were all associated with lowered levels of serotonin, cortisol, and dopamine. When serotonin levels are low, people have a decreased pain threshold and often feel depressed. During the daytime, cortisol levels remain relatively high, but dramatically drop at night. Furthermore, TL's blood pressure also drops at night, so blood circulation to his knees and ankles diminishes a lot, causing the cold and pain inside his joints. In order to maintain Professor TL's plunging blood pressure and sugar levels at night, his body automatically triggered adrenalinerelease, exacerbating his insomnia, pain, and anxiety. On the other hand, when he moved around, his blood circulation improved so his pain was reduced.

Professor TL never took any vitamins and ate very small amounts of vegetables and fruits, and too many carbohydrates, all of which contributed to his vitamin and mineral deficiency. Vitamins and minerals are critical for the sufficient functioning of the adrenal glands and the production of serotonin and other hormones. When TL was young, he ate more vegetables than meat because they were cheaper in China. When all enzyme functions declined as he got older, he could not digest the vegetables and fruit very well, so he simply stopped eating them and turned instead to carbohydrates, which could make him feel happy temporarily by increasing his blood sugar. Therefore, although his knee pain and depression responded to acupuncture quite well, his sleep did not improve much because he refused to change his diet and to take any food supplements. At last, after so many years of struggle with his knee pain, depression, and insomnia, recently he was finally convinced to eat more fruit after her granddaughter introduced him to smoothies. In this way, he can now eat two to three serving of fruit a day.

In addition, he discovered that he could sleep 5 to 6 hours without knee pain if he took a sleeping pill, which can calm down his nervous system. On the other hand, anti-inflammatory steroids never help his knee pain. This indicated that his knee pain was not caused by inflammation, but by dysfunction of his nerves. When he slept better and ate more fruits, his nerves are not so hypersensitive that when he resumed acupuncture treatments, his legs no longer jumped. Thus, I could leave the needles in even longer to calm his nervous system and his body can release more natural painkillers, endorphin and serotonin.

To the same kind of knee problem, different people suffer from different levels of pain, not always proportional to the pathological damage to the joint.

Chinese Herbal medicine and depression:

Liver Qi stagnation:

Symptoms: Irritability, depression often accompanied by anxiety, symptoms worsen under stress, chest tightness, and the tendency to sigh a lot. Symptoms temporarily relieved after taking a deep breath and after physical activities, such as walking, Qi Gong, or yoga. Intense exercise such as running more than 5 miles can induce panic attack.

Herbal formula: Chai Hu 12g, Mei Gui Hua 6g, Chuan Lian Zi 6g, Chi Shao 12g, Chuang Xiong 15g, Zhi Qiao 12g, Xiang Fu 12g, Zhi Gan Cao 6g.

Heart and Spleen deficiency:

Symptoms: Fatigue and depression do not get better after exercising or improve slightly and then worsen shortly afterwards. Insomnia, indigestion, constipation or diarrhea, pale complexion, feels cold all the time but sweats easily when doing any physical activity. Pale tongue with thin white coating and thin and weak pulse.

Herbal Formula: Zhi Huang Qi 15g, Chao Bai Zhu 12g, Xi Yang Shen 12g, Dang Gui 12g, Zhi Gan Cao 6g, Fu Shen 20g, Suan Zao Ren 20g, Sheng Jiang 6g, Da Zao 6g, Xiang Fu 12g, Long Yan Rou 6g.

Accumulated phlegm in the Middle Burner:

Symptoms: Nausea after eating greasy foods or diary products, bloating, gas. Thirsty but no desire to drink. Heavy sensation especially during humid days. Tendency to be overweight. Tongue is pale and swollen with teeth marks and thick, white, greasy coating. Pulse is slippery or soggy.

Herbal Formula: Ban Xia 6g, Chen Pi 6g, Dan Nan Xing 12g, Fu Ling 15g, Jie Geng 6g, Shi Chang Pu 12g, Yuan Zhi 12g, Dang Shen 12g, Cang Zhu 6g.

Acupuncture points for depression:

Ying Tang: at the midpoint between the two medial ends of the eyebrow.

Du20 (Bai Hui): located at the midpoint of the line connecting the apexes of the two ears.

Ci Shen Cong: 1.0 cun respectively anterior, posterior and lateral to DU 20.

HT5 (Tong Li): on the palmar aspect of the forearm, on the radial side of the tendon m. flexor carpi ulnaris, 1.0 cun above the transverse crease of the wrist.

GB8 (Shuai Gu): directly above the apex of the ears, 1.5 cun within the hairline.

CV17 (Tan Zhong): at the midpoint of the two nipples.

ST8 (Tou Wei): 4.5 cun lateral from the midline of the head, 0.5 cun above the hairline.

GB13 (Ben Shen): 0.5 cun within the anterior hairline of the forehead, 3 cun lateral to the midline of the head.

GV12 (Shen Zhu): on the posterior median line, in the depression below the spinous process of the 3rd thoracic vertebra.

Unknown point (Wu Ming Point): on the posterior median line, in the depression below the spinous process of the 2rd thoracic vertebra.

Chapter 7

Weight Gain

and Obesity

How important a health problem is weight gain in America? It is so important that First Lady Michelle Obama has made it her number one goal to end childhood obesity in one generation. One third of all American children and adolescents are obese. One third of all American adults are also obese, weighing 25% more than their ideal weight, while two thirds are overweight. It is clear that excessive weight gain has become America's new epidemic.

A behavior similar to taking drugs, smoking tobacco, or drinking alcohol, excessive eating is an addictive behavior that shortens your lifespan and is difficult to stop by force of will. Obesity increases a person's risk for developing several serious health conditions such as cardiovascular disease, hypertension, thyroid disease, polycyst ovarian syndrome, and diabetes. Every extra pound over your ideal weight may take time from your life.

Some people say to me, "Li, what do you know about weight gain, you only weigh 99 pounds?" I inwardly smile to myself because I have struggled with my weight before. Like many of us, I like food too much; I like sweets. I'm not perfect by any means but in this struggle, I am winning. I will tell you how.

What causes weight gain?

Aging: When people pass 40 years of age, their metabolic level decreases naturally. If they still eat the same amount of food as they did when they were 18, weight gain happens dramatically. Once you accumulate too much fat, your metabolic level can drop even further because fat cells cannot burn as many calories.

Hormone changes: Menopausal women have sudden drops of estrogen (50%) and progesterone (80%), which sharply decrease their metabolism. The imbalance of their estrogen and progesterone sometimes makes them crave sweets. Even if a woman eats only one cookie a day, she is adding more than 100 calories to her normal diet because she will never feel full just by eating sweets. After the sweets, she will still need the same amount of a real meal to feel satiated.

The worst thing about sweets is that most people don't know they are addictive. Because the simple sugars stimulate your brain's rewarding center, you will feel so good at that moment that you will want to have sweets every day. Sweets are even more addicting than alcohol.

When you are in your 20s, your metabolic level is high, your hormones are balanced, and you are so busy with study and work that you may forget about eating sweets. Once you reach your 40s, however, the craving for sweets becomes irresistible, especially if you are a woman with busy life. Simple sugar increases your insulin level, which quickly turns blood sugar into fat cells instead of using them to provide energy and heat. Eating sweets makes your body accumulate fat in the stomach, hip, and breast areas even though you may have slim legs and arms. Increased fat accumulation can lead to increased estrogen and sharply reduced progesterone levels so the craving snowballs.

Unhealthy diet: There is a lot of hidden sugar in processed foods and soda, which easily increases you daily caloric intake without you realizing it. You could run a marathon with all the extra calories you take in this way.

Medications: Estrogen blockers such as Tamoxifen can artificially lower your estrogen level but make you gain 30 lbs within a short period of time even if you watch your diet very carefully. This situation often happens to breast cancer patients. However, it is still important to eat healthily even when weight gain is unavoidable due to these medications because you will not have as many of the other side effects such as hot flushes, night sweats, or osteoporosis.

Hypothyroidism: If your thyroid is under-performing, you cannot produce enough heat to warm up your body or enough energy to do your daily work because your body stores the calories as fat rather than burns them to make you feel less tired and cold. An imbalanced immune system can cause your body to produce antibodies that attack your thyroid gland. A high sugar diet can also damage the thyroid by causing inflammation, which is why diabetes is always accompanied by a hypothyroid condition

Medications that lower your metabolic level: Selective serotonin reuptake inhibitors and sleeping pills can change your sleep pattern and increase your appetite because the more time you spend in deep sleep, the more your metabolism is lowered, so you gain weight gradually. When I traveled to Shanghai, I took a sleeping pill every day for 6 days and gained 5 pounds even though I walked everywhere and ate a lot of fresh vegetables and fruit and no junk food. That is why although different people may eat the same kinds of food, one person never gains weight while another tends to be chubby. If you eat healthily, being slightly chubby is not harmful for your health and may even give you more ability to cope with stress.

Alcohol: Alcohol can increase the estrogen level of men and woman and add on those empty extra calories. You may have noticed that alcoholics can have very thin arms and legs but enlarged bellies, breasts, and veins on the chest or other body areas. One CEO I knew has always followed a very healthy diet and runs religiously four times a week. He is not a big eater and only drinks two glasses of wine every day. Yet his stomach has kept on growing after turning 50 regardless of his muscular arms and legs. To resolve this problem quickly, he got an injection in his belly to dissolve the fat there. If he does not change his drinking habit, however, his fat will only re-accumulate. Furthermore, if those drugs can quickly dissolve fat tissues, just think of the damage they may cause to other organs as well.

Dehydration: Not drinking enough water can also slow down your metabolism. Please remember that every single metabolic reaction needs water as a substrate.

Birth control: Birth control pills can cause an imbalance of estrogen and progesterone and fat accumulation in your thighs, hips and breasts. If you stop taking birth control pills, you may find that you can lose 10 lbs within a short period of time.

Why do some people never gain weight even though they eat junk food or eat too much?

1. They sleep poorly or not enough: When you sleep lightly, your body burns more calories and your digestive system does not absorb nutrients as efficiently. I observed my three kids and found that two of them sleep extremely deeply and react very lethargically in the morning. The middle one, on the other hand, does not sleep as deeply so he is able to jump out of bed alert and active as soon as he opens his eyes. He probably spends more time in REM sleep. Because memory gets consolidated during REM, he remembers things very well and learns quickly. However, he never gains weight even though he eats a lot, tends to develop skin problems, and gets sick easily because he does not sleep that much.

2. Overactive sympathetic nervous system: People with overactive sympathetic nervous systems tend to produce more body heat, sweating profusely when stressed, and have a hard time settling down and relaxing. They generally sleep only 6 to 7 hours and feel bursts of the energy in the morning. Although they may be thin, they are excellent candidates for autoimmune diseases if they do not rest as needed.

3. Digestive system problems: These people may have chronic diarrhea or loose stool and tend to have bad breath. When they get

infections, they recover more slowly because their bodies cannot absorb nutrients quickly. However, if they eat sweets, they can have diarrhea and still gain weight at the same time. It is important for this group of people to gain healthy weight rather than fat tissues, so even though they are skinny, they cannot be healthy unless they eat the right foods and rest enough. Otherwise, they would be shortening the lifespan of each of their organs by using them too much and giving them too little rest.

Acupuncture and Weight Loss

Q. Wei et al.'s research on obese rats found that tryptophan and serotonin levels were decreased in certain areas of the brains in the obese group as compared to the control. Acupuncture could produce weight reduction by optimizing the serotonin (5-HT) level. Serotonin not only makes people relax and feel good, but also enhances intestinal motility to help discharge toxic materials that could produce food stagnation and internal heat. Internal heat, from a Chinese medical perspective, leads to increased appetite and more craving for food. In Western medicine, if food cannot be properly absorbed and converted into blood sugar to provide energy, it will be stored instead as fat in the body. Then, the person feels hungry all the time and must eat constantly to maintain his or her blood sugar level. It can quickly become a vicious cycle.

One way to resolve this problem is to improve digestive function by optimizing serotonin and other hormone levels so that food can be absorbed more efficiently. If people take selective serotonin reuptake inhibitor, however, they may accumulate too much serotonin in their bodies, which can dramatically increase their intestinal movement, making them so hungry that they eat constantly and gain weight. Balance is the key to achieving optimal health so letting your own body adjust its serotonin level with the help of acupuncture and dietary changes is the best way to lose weight and stay healthy.

In obese people, certain neurons in the hypothalamus (the part of the brain controlling body temperature, food intake, and other vital functions) may be less active so that they do not feel full and must continue eating until their stomachs fully expand in order to get satisfaction. Some researchers suggest that applying acupuncture to obese people may increase the excitability of the satiety center in the hypothalamus, allowing them to feel fuller on smaller amounts of food. The above mechanism has been verified in animal experiments. In 2001, a group of Chinese scientists used acupuncture to attain weight reduction in rats. They found that the activities of a group of neurons in the hypothalamus associated with the fullness sensation were markedly increased by electro acupuncture. After acupuncture treatments, the weight of the obese rats decreased and their level of serotonin as well as the activity of their ATPase, the enzyme involved in producing energy, increased. Wouldn't it be nice if you could eat less, feel good, and look better naturally with electro acupuncture?

M.T. Cabyoglu et al. of Selcuk University in Turkey suggest that acupuncture can change the activities of the auricular branch of the vagal nerve (one of the major parasympathetic nerves controlling heartbeat and digestion) and raise serotonin levels. Both of these changes have been shown to increase stomach muscle tone, thus suppressing appetite. Furthermore, when your parasympathetic nerves are more active, you feel more relaxed and crave sweets or other junk foods less.

125

Ear needling has become a widely accepted method for weight loss. Dr. D. Richard in southern Australia investigated the effects of transcutaneous electrical nerve stimulation on appetite control. Sixty overweight subjects were randomly divided into an active and a control group. The active group attached the AcuSlim machine to two ear acupuncture points twice daily for 4 weeks, whereas the control group attached the device to a part of the thumb without acupuncture points. The goal of a 2 kg weight loss was set and changes in appetite and weight were reported after four weeks. 95% of the active group noticed a suppression of appetite, whereas no one in the control group noticed such a change. None of the control group lost the required 2 kg. Both the number of subjects who lost weight and the mean weight lost were significantly higher in the active group.

While losing weight, fat tissues release a lot of toxins into the blood stream. Acupuncture helps clear up those toxins by improving your liver and kidney functions. Furthermore, electro acupuncture tones muscle and skin to prevent drooping.

Of the numerous methods we currently have for helping people control their eating, the most invasive one is the stomach bypass surgery. Even this operation can only help certain small groups of people reduce their weight. Dr. Atul Gawande, a Harvard graduate and author of the national bestseller, Complications: A Surgeon's Notes on an Imperfect Science, wrote the following story about the stomach

126

bypass surgery. One lady was able to successfully reduce her weight by more than 100 lbs after surgery. However, as time went on, she would eat a little bit more with every meal despite having severe stomachaches and vomiting afterwards. Nevertheless, she managed to eat through the pain and to re-expand her stomach to its original size, eventually gaining back all the weight she had lost.

How should we control our appetite?

1. Have you ever grabbed something to eat when you have nothing else to do? People often lose their appetite during the day when they are busy. When they get home from work, however, they tend to keep eating throughout the night while watching TV. Thus, one effective and cheap way to achieve weight loss is to read in the evening after dinner instead of sitting in front of the TV and constantly eating. Reading has the power to satisfy people with new knowledge and creative thinking, which not only helps us make great achievements, but also effectively quenches our craving for food. If you really need to watch TV, try grabbing carrot sticks instead of junk food, drink enough water, and have some relaxing tea.

2. When you eat very fast, you tend to take in more than your body needs because it takes time for the brain to sense fullness. When eating too fast, you will have already consumed too much before the signal indicating how much you have eaten reaches the brain. If you can

chew each mouthful of food 20 times, you will give the signal enough time to arrive at the brain and therefore feel satisfied with less food. Secondly, eating too fast prevents food from being properly mixed with digestive enzymes, causing indigestion.

3. How, then, can we enjoy sweets without sacrificing our health? One strategy is to eat chocolate and other sugary things right before exercising or doing other laborious work. This way, when your blood sugar suddenly spikes after consuming the sweets, your body would be able to quickly use it up. In addition, if you only eat sweets once or twice a month in moderate amounts, your body can more effectively clear the high blood sugar and you will enjoy them more than if you ate them every day.

4. Exercise can definitely help you lose weight, but you have to reach certain intensity in order to induce the endorphins needed to suppress appetite. I see people walking slowly for 30 minutes each day, which uses up blood sugar but does not tap into stored fat. At this point, your appetite actually increases due to the lowering of your blood sugar. My experience has been that when you reach your second wind, you know that your body has used up its blood sugar and stored glycogen and has started burning fat and protein. At this point, you may feel slightly nauseated, your stomach tightens up, and your appetite is suppressed. You are also quite alert for the next couple of hours because adrenaline has been released. When you attain certain intensity of

128

exercise, you no longer feel hungry and your metabolism increases dramatically for the next couple of hours.

One professional Chinese athlete used to lift weights and eat a large amount of food every day. After he stopped his regular training, he continued on the same diet and gained 150 lbs within a few years, resulting in diabetes, high blood pressure, and other medical conditions. He was determined to lose weight so he started running on the treadmill for an hour a day, which suppressed his strong appetite and burned calories. He lost most of the extra weight within a year. When he started walking instead of running, however, he gained back almost all of the weight he had lost.

My point is not that you have to run but that you need to attain high intensity exercise without hurting yourself. Still, the best way to achieve weight loss is to control how many calories you take in. Although you may feel extremely hungry when you cut down calories, exercise and acupuncture can help your body cope with the stress.

5. Eat an orange or a grapefruit two hours after your meal instead of ice cream and cookies. These two fruits can make you feel fuller with a fraction of the calories.

6. Drink some jasmine green tea two hours after your meal. The bitterness can clear your stomach heat to suppress your appetite and

stabilize your blood sugar, which is why pure tea drinkers are seldom overweight if they eat right and do not add sugar into their tea. Simple sugar bypasses the complicated digestive process so that neither tea nor smoking can stop your body from craving or absorbing it.

7. Drink 8 ounces of water half an hour before each meal and first thing in the morning to improve your digestion and increase your metabolism.

8. Stir fry bitter melon to clear your stomach heat and suppress your appetite.

9. Eat small meals more frequently to increase your metabolism.

10. Make porridge with red bean, black bean, lentil, flaxseed, and soybean in a Crockpot. You can also add vegetables to this porridge. Eat one small bowl of it before having other foods in the evening. This way, you will feel full with smaller amounts of food and your calorie intake will drop without leaving you hungry in the middle of the night.

Clinical Case Study for Weight Gain:

Martin is the CEO and founder of a biotech consulting firm located here in New England, running this company from his home office. He is a man who makes money by the strength of his mind and the great ideas it produces. With a PhD in biology, he worked for several companies and gained much experience along the way before setting up his own to help biotech companies create new products. He has no commute to work so he sits at his desk for 4 hours in the morning and 5 to 6 hours in the afternoon. Because he stays at home, he has the freedom to eat whatever he wants and whenever he wants.

Some would say that Martin has the ideal life but because he has no commute and no need to do manual labor, since starting his company, his weight gradually increased from 168 to 218 lbs over a 10 year period. By the age of 52, he was 130 lbs overweight and developed asthma. At first he thought the asthma was associated with allergies so he started using an inhaler and other medications to normalize his breathing. His level of physical activity decreased even further due to shortness of breath. Later, his otolaryngologist found a mass in his upper trachea and removed it surgically.

Initially, his breathing improved slightly but not enough to allow him to walk more than 15 minutes. However, scar tissue built up from the surgery so he had increasing difficulty breathing and eventually, his trachea would collapse when he went into deep sleep. He felt extremely tired and started losing customers because his lack of sleep was catching up to him and he could no longer produce the necessary work. His physician advised him to lose weight and to have surgery to clear his scar tissue. When winter came and the cold made his trachea contract further, his breathing became even more labored. Often, he would stop breathing in the middle of the night and had to be rushed to the hospital. This situation happened to him eight times before he came to see me for a consultation.

The first time he walked into my office, his breathing was extremely labored like he had just run up a few flights of stairs, sweat ran down his face, and looked more than a bit agitated. Only, he had not run up any stairs; he just walked the 40 feet from his car to my office on the same level.

I examined the surgical area, and to my surprise, the incision point was still open and producing pus. His tongue was dark red with a very thick, greasy yellow coating, indicating that heat and phlegm had been accumulating in his body for a long time. At this point, he had no other option but to loose weight in order to increase his lung capacity and reduce his heart burden. Because of the accumulated stomach heat, he had a very strong appetite. He loved to eat meat, especially beef, and of course sweets. However, his testosterone level was very low and his stomach could not digest food properly so it accumulated instead as fat tissue. Therefore, his blood sugar would drop shortly after he ate and soon he would have to eat again. As he gained weight, his estrogen level went up so he started losing muscle. Once his muscle to fat ratio dropped below a certain level, his metabolism decreased sharply and his body could hardly produce the required energy for him to function. Thus, he suffered from a cloudy head, fatigue, and impotence and his blood circulation was compromised. For many people with extreme weight gain, this self-perpetuating cycle happens very quickly.

I first prescribed herbs to clear his stomach heat and to eliminate the stubborn phlegm in his throat. I believed that once his phlegm was gone, his trachea would be more open despite the scar tissues and would allow him to resume rudimentary exercises. He faithfully took herbs twice a day and soon his constipation disappeared. The phlegm in his throat was reduced and gradually his breathing improved so that he could walk for 20 minutes with minimal difficulty breathing.

In the meantime, I used very strong electrical stimulation on certain points of his neck, stomach, and feet to open up his airway, tone his stomach muscle, and increase his metabolism. With improved circulation to his thyroid gland and reduced inflammation at the surgical site, his wound healed with only 4 treatments. His appetite lessened as his stomach was toned and his stomach heat reduced. After 10 treatments, he was able to walk for 40 minutes without wheezing.

He gained confidence and set a goal for him to lose more than 100 lbs, joining a weight reduction program and eating a special diet that restricted his calorie intake to 1500 a day. He continued acupuncture treatments once a week and Chinese herbs, which helped him stay on the restrictive diet, twice a day. He lost about 2 lbs every week while following the exercise regime of walking for an hour and weight lifting for another. After he lost 40 lbs, I noticed his stomach skin drooping, so I applied more electro acupuncture to tone his abdominal skin and muscle. He also developed back and leg pain because his disintegrating fat tissues released a lot of toxins that cause nerve and muscle inflammation. To treat his pain, he used Neurontin while, to heal his muscles, I used my needles. After a month, his back and leg pain were completely gone.

As soon as he stopped his diet for a few days during vacation, his weight went up within the week. After returning, he resumed Chinese herbs and acupuncture so that within two weeks, he was once again backing on track and losing weight. These treatments gave him the support he needed to stick to his diet and exercise.

All in all he lost 120 1bs within 14 months and by the end of his treatments with me, I could even see his rib cage. He could sleep through the night breathing smoothly and walk for two hours without shortness of breath. Such a wonderful accomplishment for such a wonderful man.

In this case, acupuncture helped normalize his breathing so that he could exercise and produce endorphins that allowed him cope with the stress of his low-calorie diet. Acupuncture also improved his adrenal, thyroid, and testicular functions.

There are many fad diets claiming you can lose 40 lbs within 2 months. Some dieters suffer bad side effects such as inflammation requiring hospitalization. Others successfully lose the weight as promised, but once they stop the diet, their weight quickly returns. The beauty of combining acupuncture, herbs, diet, and exercise is that it not only helps your body develop healthy eating habits but also optimizes your hormones so that your metabolism increases, your skin and muscles are toned, you have more energy and more sexual drive, and your body can discharge toxins more efficiently.

Weight loss points:

CV12: On the anterior median line of the upper abdomen, 4.0 cun above the bellybutton.

ST25: 2 cun lateral to the bellybutton.

ST8: 4.5 cun lateral from the midline of the head, .5 cun above the hairline at the corner of the forehead.

ST37: 6 cun below external knee eye, one finger-breadth (middle finger) from the anterior crest of the tibia.

ST44: on the dorsal side of the foot, located between the second and third metatarsal toes, at the junction of the red and white skin.

ST28: on the lower abdomen, 3 cun below the center of the bellybutton, 2 cun lateral to the anterior median line.

Chinese Herbal Formula for Weight Loss:

1. **Spleen deficiency with dampness and phlegm:**

Symptoms: Gains weight despite eating regular amounts of food, tends to have low thyroid function, feels cold all the time, dislikes humid weather, feels heavy all over the body, fatigued, sleeps more than 8 hours. Tongue: Pale, swollen with tooth marks, thin white coating. Pulse: Deep, soggy.

Herbal formula: Dang Shen 15g, Bai Zhu 20g, Fu Ling 20g, Yi Yi Ren 30g, Sheng Jiang 6g, Ze Xie 12g, Dan Dou Chi 12g, Huo Xiang 3g, Zhi Gan Cao 6g.

2. **Heat phlegm in the middle and lower burner:**

Symptoms: Strong appetite, eats tremendous amounts of food, often constipated, always feels warm, has bad breath, dislikes heat, sometimes suffers insomnia, sweats easily, thirsty all the time.

Tongue: Red, thick yellow greasy coating. Pulse: strong, slippery.

Herbal Formula: Zhi Zi 6g, Shi Gao 15g, Huo Xiang 6g, Zhi Mu 12g, Mai Ya 20g, Shen Qu 12g, Mu Dan Pi 6g, Yu Zhu 12g, Jing Mi 12g, Ji Nei Jin 15g

Chapter 8

Benign Prostate

Enlargement

& Prostate Cancer

There is a one in two chance that any man you meet today over 50 suffers from a prostrate issue. As the world ages, especially the Baby Boomers in the United States, men in this age group will see their bodies start having symptoms. The biggest, most common problem will be an enlarged prostate. If you are a man, this is a problem you most likely will deal with in your lifetime. This chapter will help you deal with prostrate problems, in a way that does not cause you to take powerful drugs with damaging side effects.

The prostate is a walnut-sized gland that forms part of the male reproductive system. It is made of two parts enclosed by an outer layer of tissue. The prostate is located in front of the rectum and just below the bladder. The gland surrounds the urethra, the canal through which urine passes as it exits the body. Scientists do not know all the functions of the prostate. One of its main roles, however, is to squeeze fluid into the urethra as sperms move past during sexual climax. This fluid, which makes up the semen, both energizes the sperm and makes the vaginal canal less acidic. It is common for the prostate gland to become larger as a man ages. This condition is called benign prostatic hyperplasia (BPH). In the United States in 2000, there were 4.5 million visits to physicians about prostatic enlargement.

As a man matures, the prostate goes through two main periods of growth. The first occurs early in puberty when the prostate doubles in size. Around the age of 25, the gland begins to grow again. This second growth phase often results, years later, in prostatic hyperplasia. Although the prostate continues to grow during most of a man's life, the enlargement usually doesn't cause problems until late in life. Symptoms of prostatic hyperplasia rarely appear before the age of 40, but more than half of men in their sixties and as many as 90% of those in their seventies and eighties show some symptoms. As the prostate enlarges, the layer of tissue surrounding it opposes the expansion, causing the gland to press against the urethra like a clamp on a garden hose. As a result, the bladder wall becomes thicker and more irritable. The bladder begins to contract even when it contains only small amounts of urine, increasing the frequency of urination. Eventually, the bladder weakens and loses the ability to fully empty itself, so that some of the urine remains in the bladder. The narrowing of the urethra and the partial emptying of the bladder cause many of the problems associated with prostatic hyperplasia. It has been known for many years that prostatic hyperplasia occurs mainly in older men and not at all in men whose testes were removed before puberty. For this reason, some researchers believe that factors related to aging and the testes may spur the development of prostatic hyperplasia. However, if removing the testes before puberty prevents prostate enlargement because it results in low testosterone, then aging, which also decreases testosterone, should not lead to the enlargement of the prostate. Therefore, there must be other factors involved. The new research shows that estrogen can stimulate prostate growing. Doctors now use an estrogen blocker to treat prostate cancer after surgery, in order to prevent prostate cancer cell growth.

What causes prostatic hyperplasia?

1. Diabetes inflames blood vessels, causing inflammation of the prostate.

2. Obesity can lead to higher levels of estrogen in men, stimulating prostate growth.

3. An abnormality may happen during the second period of prostate growth, around the age of twenty.

4. Dihydrotestosterone (DHT), a substance derived from the testosterone in the prostate, adrenal glands, testes and hair follicles, stimulates prostatic growth. Some research suggests that, even with the drop in the level of blood testosterone, older men continue to produce and accumulate high levels of dihydrotestosterone in the prostate. This accumulation may encourage the growth of prostate cells. Scientists have also noted that men who do not produce dihydrotestosterone do not develop prostatic hyperplasia.

5. Regular alcohol consumption compromises liver function, so that the liver cannot deactivate estrogen and dihydrotestosterone effectively, leading to increased levels of estrogen and thus the enlargement of the prostate.

6. Tensile strength of the prostate capsule: If the capsule outside the prostate loses its elasticity, the enlarged prostate will not be able to grow outwards. Instead, the gland will compress the urethra, causing more irritation. For the same amount of prostate enlargement, a man with a stretchy prostate capsule will not suffer the severe urination problems that a man without one will experience. Deficiency of vitamin C may cause this dysfunction of the prostate capsule and other connective tissues.

7. High dosage of fish oil: One study from the National Cancer Institute indicates that men who take a high dosage of flaxseed or fish

oil for a long time have a greater risk of getting prostate cancer or prostate enlargement. Too much Omega-3 may influence the hormone balance.

Symptoms of prostatic hyperplasia

Many symptoms of prostatic hyperplasia stem from the obstruction of the urethra and the gradual loss of bladder function, which results in the incomplete emptying of the bladder. Although the symptoms of prostatic hyperplasia vary, the most common ones involve problems with urination, such as a hesitant, interrupted, or weak stream, an urgency to urinate, leaking or dribbling, and more frequent urination, especially at night.

The size of the prostate does not always determine how severe the obstruction of the urethra or the symptoms will be. Some men with greatly enlarged prostates have little obstruction and fewer symptoms, whereas others with less enlarged glands have more blockage and severe problems. Symptoms are associated with bladder and urethra function as well. If you already have compromised bladder function due to diabetes, neuropathy, or high blood pressure, as well as bladder and urethra inflammation, your symptoms tend to be more severe. If living long enough, almost all men will develop prostate enlargement, but only 50% will have clinical symptoms. The above reasons may explain why other 50% of men have very limited urination problems. I treated a 91-year-old graduate of MIT who could still sleep for 6 to 8 hours without getting up to urinate. It is highly likely that, at 91 years of age, this gentleman has an enlarged prostate. Because he has lived a healthy lifestyle, however, he does not have too much inflammation in his blood vessels, prostate, or bladder and therefore shows no symptoms.

Medications may also play a role in the development of clinical symptoms. Sometimes, a man may not know that he has an obstruction until he suddenly finds himself unable to urinate at all. Taking over-the-counter cold or allergy medications may trigger this condition, called acute urinary retention. Such medications contain a decongestant drug known as a sympathomimetic. One potential side effect of sympathomimetics is the interruption of the normal function of bladder and urethra, suddenly preventing the patient from urinating. Alcohol, cold temperatures, or a long period of immobility can also cause urinary retention. Urinary retention and the resulting strain on the bladder may lead to urinary tract infections, bladder or kidney damage, bladder stones, and incontinence (the inability to control urination). If the bladder is permanently damaged, treatment for prostatic hyperplasia may be ineffective. Therefore, receiving instant medical attention for urinary retention is very important for preventing permanent damage to the bladder.

How to prevent urinary problems

1. Apply heat to the lower abdominal area if the bladder cannot relax or contract normally.

2. Build stronger pelvic muscles to control the bladder by squeezing them as if you were trying to stop urine flow. Each set of this exercise includes 10 seconds of contraction and 10 of relaxation. Do 10 to 20 sets daily.

3. Apply moxa on CV4 (on the midline of the abdomen, 3 cun below the umbilicus), CV3 (on the midline of the abdomen, 4 cun below the umbilicus), and Kid5 (1 cun directly below Kid3 in the depression between the medial malleolus and the tendon calcaneus, at the same level as the tip of the medial malleolus).

4. Drink plenty of water to prevent bladder infections.

5. Cut down on or completely stop alcohol intake.

6. Get acupuncture or acupressure to strengthen the bladder muscles and to regenerate the function of the nerves to control the bladder.

7. Avoid long term usage of decongestant medications if you already experience difficulty urinating. Instead, you can use an herbal remedy to fix your cold, allergy or even flu.

8. Do not hold your urine for too long, which over-stretches the bladder muscles, causing weakness of the muscle.

Clinical Case Study for Prostate Problems

DK is everyman. When I first met him I thought he seemed depressed or at least low energy. He appeared calm, walked with the gate of a former athlete, but his face told me that underneath, he was somehow irritated or disappointed in something. He was friendly enough as I began my intake.

DK had high blood pressure and high cholesterol, so he had been taking Lipitor and a blood pressure medication for more than five years. When he first started taking the blood pressure medication, he developed impotence; his beautiful wife thought he might not be interested in her anymore. After mentioning this problem to his physician, he tried many different kinds of blood pressure medications until he finally found one that allowed him to keep his sexual function. Occasionally, if his stress level became too high, he would develop temporary impotence.

His major complaints, however, were muscle pain on his upper and lower back and prostate problems. Because his muscle pain always occurred at the same spot, it indicated that there was some kind of chronic inflammation in the area instead of just a muscle sprain. Interestingly, swimming did not help the pain at all, even though he would feel very relaxed afterwards. Every time he received acupuncture for muscle pain, he felt better, but the pain always returned shortly afterwards. It seemed that there was an underlying problem causing those muscle aches. I suspected that Lipitor was the underlying problem, but because DK really enjoyed eating sweets, he was not willing to change his diet and would rather continue taking Lipitor to lower his cholesterol.

At the age of 55, he was diagnosed with prostatic hyperplasia when he suddenly could not urinate after coming back from a vacation. He was rushed to an emergency room where a catheter was put into his bladder. The urologist said that his prostate enlargement was moderate, which would not cause urination problems for most other people. When DK was very young, however, he worked in a very remote area without a restroom close by, so he used to hold his urine for many hours during the day. Of course, he could not drink much water. The first factor may have caused his bladder muscles to lose their elasticity after many years of over-stretching; furthermore, the lack of water intake may have led to a urinary tract infection. As a result of his weakened bladder muscles, he suffered from urinary retention.

One time, while traveling, DK sat in an airplane for a long time after taking a cold medication. All of a sudden, his bladder muscles stopped functioning. Because acute urinary retention had happened to him many times, DK finally decided to deal with the problem. I started acupuncture treatments on his lower abdominal and back areas. When he had constipation, his urinary retention got worse, with increased urination frequency and urgency. One time, the Chinese herbal formula that I gave him dramatically improved his urination and constipation when he was on a vacation in Mexico. However, because he continued taking his blood pressure medication, which influences his bladder muscles, the problem returned periodically.

Finally, he became convinced that using laser surgery to abrade off part of his prostate might be the only way to solve his problem. He assumed that if his problems were due to an enlarged prostate, the frequent urination and urine retention should be fixed after the surgery. Following the protocol, he had a catheter inserted during and after surgery. Because his bladder muscles became even weaker with the catheter, he could not urinate for a while after surgery, and the frequency of urination increased. I told him that his bladder muscles needed be strengthened so that he could empty his bladder more efficiently and prevent infection. He completed 10 acupuncture treatments after his catheter was removed, and he could urinate by himself normally after just one treatment. For a couple of years after the surgery, his constant urge to urinate was reduced by acupuncture treatments once or twice a month. With strengthened bladder muscles, the amount of residual urine in his bladder was dramatically reduced. The urgency of his desire to urinate also decreased due to the lessened inflammation of his bladder and urethra. He continued taking all of his medications and receiving acupuncture treatments for many years. His tongue, however, often showed a thick greasy coating, indicating digestive inefficiency, which can cause urinary problems. Therefore, I used herbs to improve his digestion.

After the surgery, his physician had put him on diazepam to reduce his anxiety. His impotence got worse as a side effect of the drug. In the ensuing treatment, I focused on improving his testosterone level and erectile function. Finally, he stopped taking diazepam and flomax, a commonly used medication to relax the bladder muscles. With continuing acupuncture treatments, his impotence was gone. Ten months after his prostate surgery, he had another attack of acute urinary retention in June of 2002. I gave him 10 acupuncture treatments to bring back his urination.

Acupuncture helped restore his normal urinary function every time the problem was triggered by stress, cold, or other conditions. In June of 2005, DK developed kidney stones. The pain was so severe that he vomited bile and almost fainted once. He told me that he drank tea all day long because he thought that the more antioxidants he had, the better. I have been treating this gentleman for more than 6 years now and I did not see any dramatic improvements after the laser surgery on his prostate; he still has acute urinary retention once or twice a year. Sometimes, he has even urinated blood, which scared him to death at first. I think that if he stopped eating so much simple sugar and lowered his cholesterol by changing his lifestyle and cut down on his medications, he could improve his bladder function. Stress was another trigger that aggravated his urinary problem. One time, when he needed to fast for 24 hours in order to take a blood test, his urinary retention instantly returned. His urinary problem has not yet been completely solved.

What causes increased mortality of prostate cancer?

1. High insulin level: Demetrius Albanes, M.D., of the Nutritional Epidemiology Branch, Division of Cancer Epidemiology and Genetics at the National Cancer Institute in Bethesda, Md., and colleagues conducted a prospective case–cohort study nested within a cancer prevention study of Finnish men (100 case subjects with prostate cancer and 400 non-case subjects without prostate cancer). Levels of insulin were determined in fasting serum that had been collected 5-12 years before diagnosis of prostate cancer. The results indicated that higher blood insulin levels, even within the normal range, are associated with increased risk of prostate cancer. Even if you don't have diabetes, if you eat chocolate (unless it is 90% cocoa) or other sweets every day, your insulin level will surge every time you put this magic food into you mouth, and eventually you will develop insulin resistance. By that time, your body has to produce more insulin in order to lower the blood sugar level because the normal level of insulin does not work anymore. High insulin causes more inflammation, which can lead to prostate cancer

2. Increased estrogen levels in alcoholics: even if you have just one glass of red wine every day, you can develop two problems:

Your liver function can become compromised, so that it will not clear up estrogen efficiently. Higher levels of estrogen will make men develop bigger breasts, dilated small blood vessels, loose muscle and an enlarged prostate.

Alcohol can increase the activity of aromatase, an enzyme in charge of converting testosterone into estrogen.

3. Zinc deficiency can increase the activity of aromatase, so men with this condition may produce more estrogen.

4. Old age: By the age of eighty, most men develop prostate cancer, but they do not usually die of prostate cancer. The later the prostate cancer develops, the slower the growth of the cancer because of lowered levels of several hormones.

5. A study at Harvard indicated that too much flax seed or fish oil can increase the prostate cancer rate, but taking flax seed instead of flaxseed oil would be a better choice because there is a lower concentration of omega-3.

How can you improve your rate of survival from prostate cancer?

Dr. Jing Ma and his colleagues in Harvard Medical School looked at information on more than 2,500 men who had been followed for 24 years after they were diagnosed with prostate cancer. The research indicated that overweight men (those with a BMI of 25 to 29) had a 47 percent higher risk of dying from prostate cancer, while obese men (BMI of 30 or over) were more than two-and-a-half times more likely to die of the disease, compared with men of healthy weight (BMI under 25). Men with the highest concentrations of C-peptide (a marker of insulin levels in the blood) also had more than double the risk of dying from their cancer compared with men having the lowest levels. Finally, men who had a BMI of more than 25 *and* high C-peptide concentrations had quadruple the risk of dying from prostate cancer compared with men who had lower BMIs and lower C-peptide levels.

How to prevent prostate cancer or live with prostate cancer?

Weight loss: aromatase, an enzyme, which stimulates the body to produce more estrogen, resides in fat cells. The less fat you have, the less aromatase and estrogen you have.

Lower levels of insulin: exercise can make you body becomes more sensitive to the effects of insulin. The more muscle you have, the less insulin you need when you eat carbohydrates or sweets, and the more calories you can burn.

Flavonoids can inhibit aromatase, so that your body will produce less estrogen with those natural aromatase inhibitors. Flavonoid can be found in the herb Passiflora incarnate (Purple Passion Flower); in some fruits and vegetables such as cabbage, onions/garlic and apples; in parsley, celery, and chamomile; and in soy.

Acupuncture and prostate function:

UB26: On the back, 1.5 cun lateral to the lower border of the spinous process of the 5th lumbar vertebra.

UB28: 0.5 cun lateral to the middle sacral crest, at the level of the 2nd posterior sacral foramen.

CV3: On the anterior median line of the lower abdomen, 4 cun below the umbilicus.

Du4: on the posterior median line, in the depression below the spinous process of the 2nd lumbar vertebra.

UB32: in the 2nd sacral foramen.

CV4: On the anterior median line of the lower abdomen, 3 cun below the umbilicus.

Moxa:

Kid1: On the sole, in the depression when the foot is in plantar flexion, approximately at the anterior third and the posterior two thirds of the line from the web between the 2nd and 3rd toes to the back of the heel.

CV3: On the anterior median line of the lower abdomen, 4 cun below the umbilicus.

Dong Shi Qi Xue:

Hai Bao: between SP1 and SP3.

Mu Fu: 0.3 cun lateral to the midline of the second toe in the middle of the second joint.

Ma Kuai Shui: 4 fen below SI18

Shen Guan: 1.5 inches below SP9.

Ear Needle: Kidney, Urine Bladder, Nao Dian, Pi Zhi Xia

Chinese Herbs and enlarged prostate:

1. Damp heat in lower burner with blood stasis:

Enlarged prostate, abdominal pain, dribbling urination, dry mouth, and tendency to drink a lot of water. Tongue: red, thin yellow greasy coating, Pulse: slippery.

Herbal formula: Chao Zhi Mu 9g, Chao Huang Bai 9g, Sheng Ma 9g, Rou Gui 0.9g, Shi Wei 15g, Ju Mai 15g, Dang Shen 30g, Dang Gui 12g, Chao Chi Shao 12g, Hai Zao 12g, Hu Zhang 18g, Hua Shi 18g, Hu Po Mo 1.2g, Shu Da Huang 15g.

2. Damp heat with kidney Yin deficiency:

Enlarged prostate, difficulty to urinate, urine stream like thread, or no urine at all, lower back is weak and sore, light headed with ear ringing, heat sensation in the palm and bottom of the feet, Tongue: red with little coating or greasy coating, Pulse: thin, fast.

Herbal formula: Shu Di 30g, Shan Yao 30g, Shan Yu Rou 15g, Hua Shi 15g, Qing Dai 15, Niu Xi 15g, Fu Ling 12g, Liu Ji Nu 12g, Ze Xie 10g, Dan Pi 10g, Che Qian Zi 10g, Bian Xu 20g, Ju Mai 20g, Gan Cao 6g, Deng Xin Cao 3g.

3. Kidney Yang deficiency with lung and spleen qi deficiency:

Enlarged prostate, difficulty to urinate, urine stream like thread, urine retention, weak lower back and joint, aversion to cold, shortness of breath, fatigue, Tongue: pale with teeth marks, Pulse: deep thin and weak.

Herbal formula: Rou Cong Rong 20g, Suo Yang 20g, Tu Si Zi 20g, Wang Bu Liu Xing 15g, Huang Qi 15g, Chuan Niu Xi 20g, Yi Mu Cao 20g.

Patterned Herbs: Jin Gui Shen Qi Wan, Suo Quan Wan, Jin Suo Gu Jing Wan.

Chapter 9

The Embarrassing Problem of Excessive

Sweating

I have always had a soft spot in my heart for people who have problems such as sweating excessively. This kind of problem makes you suffer in two ways: socially and physically. These people always feel like everyone is looking at them. It is a difficult problem to deal with socially, and it really affects how you feel about yourself. What can you do about it? If you consult your doctor, he might suggest surgery. This might solve the problem instantly, but maybe it's not your best first option, considering the side effects, which include problems such as extremely dry skin around the face, neck and scalp, sweaty face upon eating or randomly smelling certain kinds of foods, lowered heart rate, excessive sweating from the waist down, or weakness or paralysis of the upper arm. Not everyone experiences these side effects, but some do. Before you decide to go for surgery, do your research and find out the success rates and the long-term effects. You might also consider a less invasive approach. Let me tell you about a patient of mine with this condition whom I treated using techniques based upon Traditional Chinese Medicine and a hearty dose of common sense.

Harvey Bryce had suffered from excessive sweating since his early childhood. When I treated him, at 40 years of age, he had been living with this difficult problem for over three decades. Little did his wife and two young children know that this problem caused him frustration and social awkwardness. He had begun his own plumbing business and tried to work closely with his customers. Secretly, he always felt he needed to stand off from them physically and also . . . emotionally. It was something he always wished he could change about himself. The sweats were mostly located in his hands, armpits, chest, abdomen, and groin and buttocks area. When he reached 40 years of age, the sweating had become so severe that he would find himself watching TV in a regular temperature room when suddenly the waterworks would start. The frequency and intensity had recently become worse and worse. He didn't know what to do or to whom to turn.

As I talked with him about his life, he seemed normal enough. I noted that he usually had red wine every night at dinner and coffee in the morning. Every night, after his children went to bed, he would eat a little pastry that he greatly enjoyed. He noticed that after eating some foods, especially spicy or warm food, drinking coffee or wine, getting excited about something or even just laughing hard, his excessive sweating might be triggered. If he became nervous about sweating, he would sweat even more with the anxiety. It seemed that he had everything to fear including fear itself. So I began my investigation.

During my intake evaluation, when I looked at his tongue, the coating was very thick and greasy at the back, with cracks in the middle, indicating that his digestion was not optimal. He told me that he tended to over-think problems and situations to the point that it would consume his thoughts. His blood pressure was slightly above the normal range. And, like many introverted people, he never enjoyed being in a crowd; in fact, it made him a bit uneasy. What he really loved was to focus on his own job in a quiet environment.

Now I really had my antenna up. It came out in conversation that he tended to eat a lot but did not gain weight. When other people watched him eating, they were surprised that he was so fit and in such great shape considering how much he ate. This fact was a major clue to me into what was going on with his condition. Once he started exercising, his sweating would spike to the point that he would be drenched. The unusual thing was that both of his hands would sweat and become very cold at the same time. Hmmm . . .

So what did this all mean? Why was this happening to such a nice, caring man? How could I help him get out of this miserable situation? I thought that I should employ my two ultra-sophisticated diagnostic instruments: cutting edge scientific research mated with medical theory first documented in 475 BC and improved through the ages: Traditional Chinese Medicine (TCM), an unbeatable duo!

What causes excessive sweating (hyperhidrosis)?

We needed to investigate what was known in medical science research literature about this smelly, wet, embarrassing condition. First, we know that excessive sweating is caused by over-active sweat glands. The sweat gland is controlled by branches of sympathetic nerves in the chest area, which are controlled by the hypothalamus, a part of the brain controlling appetite, body temperature, thirst, fatigue, anger and circadian cycles. Whew, that's a lot to remember, and complicated. People suffering from this condition can sweat spontaneously, even at room temperature, and excessively in a slightly warm environment. The most common parts of the body that sweat are the palms, feet, armpits, chest, abdominal area and face. Unfortunately, those who sweat excessively tend to have a special body odor, so that they smell bad, another thing to be self-conscious about.

If you have this problem, you can most likely blame your parents, because genetic make-up plays a big part. People with very

159

sensitive sympathetic nervous systems tend to have hyperhidrosis, and very sensitive nervous systems tend to run in the family. Thus, you may have inherited your mom's problems, but you don't have to accept them. You can return that bad hand you've been dealt and get a much better one, so don't worry.

But you've got to do some work yourself. There are life style choices you can make that will lessen this problem or possibly make it go away completely. You can make decisions that will change things. Start by not drinking so much alcohol, which can intensify the symptoms. Alcohol can produce a lot of heat inside your body and get your nervous system going. In order to maintain a normal body temperature, you have to expel extra heat through sweat and urination. That is why people tend to drink more alcohol in cold weather. Alcoholics tend to have clammy hands and feet and often look like Santa with a red face. There are cases where people never had this problem growing up, only to have it appear later in life, usually triggered by drinking too much alcohol. So, please back off the drinks, for your own health, dignity and peace of mind. You don't have to stop completely, just reduce, reduce, and reduce until your problem goes away.

Other things that stimulate your nervous system that you can reduce:

1. Caffeine stimulates your sympathetic nerves, so your body becomes even more sensitive to temperature changes.

2. Warm drinks and food can make you sweat more.

3. Low and high blood sugar levels can induce adrenaline release to intensify sweating.

4. Stress can induce cortisol and adrenaline release to stimulate the nervous system.

5. Multi-tasking: when you do three things at the same time, your body has to release more adrenaline, which stimulates the nervous system.

6. Imbalanced progesterone and estrogen also sensitizes your nervous system, so that your body may react very strongly to small temperature changes. That is why menopausal women sweat easily, then quickly feel chilled afterwards. Men who use testosterone cream for a long time tend to sweat a lot with a special body odor.

7. Obesity: Obese people have higher levels of cortisol and estrogen. They can tolerate stress better than skinny people, but they have less tolerance for heat. When obese women go through menopause, they have more hot flashes than average-weight women.

8. Spicy foods also produce internal heat. People can tolerate spicy foods in a very damp and cold climate, but if they leave for warmer places, they have to change their eating habits accordingly.

My Diagnosis: What did I tell Harvey?

Now I had to make my diagnosis. I must help my long-suffering patient. All of these symptoms indicated that Harvey Bryce had a very active sympathetic nervous system, which could very easily go into action, producing a lot of heat. His basal body temperature was around 98 degrees, indicating a higher starting metabolic level. The hyperactive nervous system also caused his blood pressure to go up and down with a high degree of variability.

I put all the symptoms together and confronted him with the facts and suggested that he eliminate all the possible triggers. I told him to start cutting down his pastry to every other night and reduce from three cups of coffee to two cups, only in the morning. Unfortunately, he was not willing to cut down his red wine. It was very difficult for him to change this habit, and I know it is one of the most difficult changes to make. I was told by one of my close friends and advisors that if I can convince all the alcoholics to give up alcohol, I will win the Nobel prize! The good thing was that I didn't have an alcoholic patient, only someone who likes wine a bit too much for his own health. Therefore, I added acupuncture and herbs to make the transition easier.

How Did Harvey Do?

During acupuncture treatment, Harvey's body produced more relaxing chemicals such as endorphins, serotonin, and GABA to cope with his stress. One of the reasons he loved to eat pastry every night was that sweets could help induce endorphins to make him feel better. However, after eating all these comfort foods, his blood sugar would go up the next morning. This in turn would cause the sympathetic nervous system to become over sensitive. Then he would drink a couple of cups of coffee, which would stimulate his nervous system even more. Oh boy, see how this works; this is constant bombardment of his sensitive nervous system. How could he not be in trouble? His imbalanced nervous system also became over sensitized, because of constant work stress during the daytime, a very bad cycle to be caught in. Eventually this cycle would cause Harvey to sweat spontaneously.

After 10 treatments, I asked him to cut down his coffee from two cups to one. Within a month, he noticed that his spontaneous sweating lessened. Furthermore, after exercising, the duration and intensity of sweating were reduced. He was starting to see the light at the end of the tunnel, and that made him work all the harder to get better. After taking his herbal formula for a month, his tongue coating became thinner on the front half of his tongue. His seasonal allergies were reduced; He felt calmer and had a slightly increased bowel movement, which also helped to discharge the extra heat from his body. And as a bonus, he lost 10 pounds without any special diet, especially the belly fat. How wonderful! He and I were ecstatic!

How did he progress from there? Three months after acupuncture treatment, he was drinking only one cup of coffee and eating a pastry only once or twice a week, during the weekend when he had more physical exercise that enabled his blood sugar to be lowered quickly. However, cutting down red wine continued to be extremely difficult, even though he knew that alcohol would induce the sweating and damage his liver function. I told him that he could try acupuncture and Chinese herbal medicine to see if his sweating could be controlled with routine alcohol intake, but that changing this habit might shorten the treatment time.

He also noticed that his five-year-old son had a similar sweating problem. I would assume that, at this young age, his son did not drink alcohol or coffee, but he did eat a lot of sweets, as do other American children. He was a talented kid, with so much energy that he could hardly sit down. His fight or flight system was so active that any stressful condition would trigger the problem.

He came to my office on a Tuesday and said, "Li, I now have a drink only on the weekend, once during my Saturday dinner. It is a special occasion for my wife and me, so we celebrate with wine. Slowly, Harvey improved from there, and within three months his problem had vanished. All the work he had done to improve had finally taken effect. That last commitment to reduce wine intake was the nail in the coffin for his periodic sweats. I asked him what caused him to decide to reduce his wine. At this point, he said, "My son has this problem as well, Li; I want to lead him to a better life, and what better way than to show him by example." Thus, in the end, Harvey got better. He also noticed that he could now deal with difficult situations much more calmly and wisely even though his stress level is extremely high with the bad economy. He got better because he cared so much for the quality of his life and the life of his young son.

Bring This to Your Traditional Chinese Medicine Doctor

HT5: the point is located on the radial side of the tendon of m. flexor carpi ulnaris, 1 cun above the transverse crease of the wrist.

LI 11: When the elbow is flexed, the point is in the depression at the lateral end of the transverse cubital crease, midway between LU 5 and the lateral epicondyle of the humerus.

SI7: located on the dorsal ulnar aspect of the forearm, 5 cun above the transverse crease of the wrist, on the line connecting SI 5 (On the dorsal ulnar aspect of the forearm, right on the wrist line), and SI 8 (On the medial aspect of the elbow, in the depression between the olecranon of the ulna and the medial epicondyle of the humerus).

UB44: located on the back, 3.0 cun lateral to the lower border of the spinous process of the 5th thoracic vertebra.

UB45: located on the back, 3.0 cun lateral to the lower border of the spinous process of the 6th thoracic vertebra.

PC6: located on the palmar aspect of the forearm, 2 cun above the transverse crease of the wrist, between the tendons of m. palmaris longus and m. flexor carpi radialis.

HT1: located at the apex of the axillary fossa, where the axillary artery pulsates.

Chinese Herbal Medicine to restore the balance of your nervous system:

1. **Food Stagnation with excessive heat in the stomach**: very common due to overeating, ice cold drinks and anti-acid medication: If food is not properly digested, it will become toxin, producing heat.

Symptoms: strong appetite all the time, bloating, gas, bad breath, smelly stool, sweating located mainly in chest, abdominal, groin area and armpit, with clammy palms. Tongue coating is very thick and greasy, especially at the back of the tongue. Pulse is slippery or forceful.

166

Self-healing:

Cut down or stop alcohol intake

Have small, more frequent meals

Barley tea or barley green tea 2 times a day

Do not drink too much coffee because caffeine will stimulate insulin release, lowering your sugar faster, so that you feel hungry all the time.

Soak orange peel in hot water and drink twice a day.

Drink water two hours after meal, or half an hour before meal.

One teaspoon apple cider vinegar twice a day; after symptoms get better, then cut down to once a day.

Decrease simple sugar intake, have at least one apple per day.

Chinese Herbal Formula: Lian Zi 12g, Chao Mai Ya 15g, Jiao Shan Zha 20g, Fu Ling 12g, Bai Zhu 12g, Fu Xiao Mai 30g, Shi Gao 15g, Chi Shao 15g, Fang Feng 6g.

Acupuncture Points:

CV12: located on the front midline, 4 inches above the belly button.

CV11: located on the front midline, 5 inches above the belly buttons.

ST43: located on the dorsal part of the feet, in the depression distal to the junction of the second and third metatarsal bones.

2. Kidney Yin deficiency with heat:

Symptoms: Loss of hair in early thirties, skinny, night sweats, increasing sweat when excited, sweating mostly in the palms, not much on the feet, dry skin in some areas, sweating more when doing multi-tasking, constant tiredness with quick recovery from nap. Sleep can be interrupted if thinking too much.

Self healing techniques:

Decrease spicy food

Drink enough water, at least half of your weight in fluid ounces.

Eat more sour tasting food, which can generate more Yin (body fluids) in your body.

Have wild yam every other day

Do not eat too many nuts

Alcohol only every other week or during holiday seasons

No Ginseng tea or any kind of stimulant that dries up body's fluids

Add Lycium seed into your soup twice a week

Watermelon, cranberries, or blueberries twice a week

Well-cooked red beans 3 times a week.

Avoid long-term usage of anti-histamine, anti-depression, or diuretic medications

Acupressure

Kid2: anterior and inferior to the medial malleolus, in the depression on the lower border of the tuberosity of the navicular.

Ht6: when the palm faces upward, the point is on the radial side of the tendon of m. flexor carpi ulnaris, 0.5 cun above the transverse crease of the wrist.

Herbal Formula: He Shou Wu 6g, Nu Zhen Zi 9g, Mo Han Lian 9g, Zhi Zi 6g, Zhi Mu 6g, Shan Yao 12g, Huang Jing 15g, Fu Ling 12g, Sheng Bai Zhu 12g, Sheng Di 12g, Mu Dang Pi 6g.

Acupuncture points:

Kid8: located 2 cun directly above Kid3 (between the medial malleolus and Achilles tendons), 0.5 cun anterior to Kid7, posterior to the medial border of the tibia.

Kid2: located on the medial aspect of the foot, below the tuberosity of the navicular bone, at the junction of the red and white skin.

UB26: 1.5 cun lateral to the lower border of the spinous process of the 5th lumbar vertebra.

3. **Excessive heat in lung or heart due to over-thinking or energy blockage in upper burner:**

Symptoms: sweating mainly in the palms and upper body, thinking and planning all the time, compulsive thinking if a person has too much free time, waking up at 3 or 4 am and can not fall back to sleep, dry throat, dry coughing, palpitation sometimes.

Self-healing techniques:

Meditation with deep breathing twice a day for 15 min. each time

Have some bitter melon, or drink green tea to clear the upper burner heat.

Stretching exercises two hours before going to sleep to calm the nervous system.

Do not do exercises intensely.

Practicing Qi Gong.

Acupuncture once a week if the above methods can not balance your nervous system.

When your mind is stuck, divert your attention by reading an interesting book or doing sewing or gardening.

Herbal Formula: Zhi Zi 6g, Dan Dou Chi 6g, Sheng Di 6g, Suan Zao Ren 12g, Zhu Ye 6g, Lian qiao 9g, Zhen Zhu Mu 15g, Mu Li 15g, Chai Hu 6g

Acupuncture points:

UB43: On the back, 3.0 cun lateral to the lower border of the spinous process of the 4th thoracic vertebra.

UB44: On the back, 3.0 cun lateral to the lower border of the spinous process of the 5th thoracic vertebra.

Excess sweating point: 1.5 inch below SI13 (In the region of the scapula, on the medial extremity of the suprascapular fossa).

Kid2: On the medial aspect of the foot, below the tuberosity of the navicular bone, at the junction of the red and white skin.

Chapter Ten

Low Testosterone

It was a cool night. My husband and I had been invited to a neighborhood party in my hometown of West Roxbury, Massachusetts. Many friends of my daughter and their parents attended an outside spring barbeque. As with many of my patients, I met this one by chance. A brief introduction by the host led from one topic to another. This man and his wife, Bill and Julie Rosenthal, both in their fifties and in good shape, talked about their yoga regime, which sounded as if they were dedicated to keeping fit and healthy. I talked about my practice and the kinds of issues that I typically treated. Of the two, I could see that he was interested but had reservations. He was a man of few words; he spoke more with facial expression. However, I could tell by looking at him that he had a condition that he was unwilling to talk about. I didn't know exactly what it was. I spoke with many people that night and didn't think much more about it.

A few weeks later, Mr. Rosenthal appeared in my waiting room without an appointment. I had a very full patient load that day, so it was difficult to make time for his questions, but I tried my best between visits to answer his halting queries. He did not reveal much about himself, but his questions centered around energy levels or something like that. I think I was more confused about his issues when he left. My confusion was not long-lived because I received a call the following week to set up an appointment.

My first appointment takes longer than subsequent visits because it is here that I gain insight into my patients. I ask questions and observe. There are many clues that I search for that first time. I am seeing, listening, feeling for answers beyond the words that my patients use to describe their symptoms.

Mr. Rosenthal asked to make an appointment for the following week. The day of his appointment, I had him fill out a detailed questionnaire concerning general health issues. Sometimes patients will identify problems here that they have not talked about. We all live with issues that we don't like to speak about and are more comfortable expressing in writing. He identified at that time that he had knee pain and stomach problems.

At his intake appointment, I learned that beyond stomach cramps and knee pain, he suffered from panic attacks periodically. He told me that he had a high stress managerial position in a high-tech company and that he felt a bit out of control on occasion. I understood generally what he was telling me; however, I could tell at that point that he had other health problems that he didn't feel comfortable sharing. By his manner and my physical observations, I was convinced he had not told me the full story.

As I treated him further, I found out more. He had been a serious runner all his life and had had arthritis in his knee for going on 10 years. Stomach issues since childhood plagued him. Whenever he skipped a meal or got nervous about something, he would have severe stomach pain. He mentioned that recently he had developed rashes on his torso. At the fifth visit, I found out what he had been unwilling to talk about. He was too reserved a man and so much a product of his socially conservative New England upbringing.

He had told me that he had never shared this with anyone else, not even his wife.

Early in his fifties, he noticed that his high sex drive was gone. It depressed him, and caused him to lose energy in a general way. He went to see his urologist and found out that his testosterone level was down at the lower end of the normal range. He started testosterone cream externally, hoping to save his libido and improve the quality of his sex life. With his stressful daily job, he could not sleep very well and developed night sweats and dizziness.

What Were Mr. Rosenthal's Problems?

When I first met Mr. Rosenthal, he mentioned that he always felt hot at room temperature and was constantly sweating. He drank wine in moderation, maybe a glass with dinner each night. He was not sleeping well.

I started clearing his blocked heat in his upper and lower body using acupuncture. After only three treatments, his stomach problems affected him less frequently, while he continued his herbal powder from a naturopathic doctor. His panic attacks lessened, and his knee pain abated. After another three treatments, he could have lunch with business partners without worrying about his stomach cramps. His sleep, although not perfect, was improving. I was very surprised by his quick response and thought that maybe he was on a tight budget, so we cut down his treatments to once a month. It seemed that the once a month treatment was able to help his body optimize the digestive function. He mentioned that his sleep could be interrupted by his alcohol intake. After five treatments, he got his testosterone retested: it had almost doubled. In the mean time, he had more spontaneous sweating with increased blood pressure. I suggested that he cut down his testosterone gel to every other day. During the summer, his blood pressure decreased with reduced testosterone gel, and his face was not as red as before.

In November, I treated him twice with neck and back points, while he laid face-down, to relieve his tightness in those areas. He could then sleep for 6 straight hours. He maintained monthly treatments, and gradually his sleep became deeper and lasted for seven hours sometimes.

When the economy started to dive in 2008, his testosterone dropped to 6 (normal is above 9) when his stress level was increased, even with very good sleep. He increased the testosterone dosage to save his libido again. I suggested that he switch to bioidentical testosterone if he had to use hormones. His sleep would be improved to seven hours right after acupuncture treatment but gradually went back to five hours within two weeks. He then increased the frequency of treatments to every two weeks. Surprisingly, his old allergies came back, and he could not lie face-down to have back treatment. He mysteriously stopped treatments for a month; I figured he might have some other issues.

When he finally called a month after his last treatment in October, he reported that he had developed eye tearing right after the last acupuncture treatment. His left eye had turned red, with tears coming down the face, especially in the morning. His left eye was also constantly producing pus. Afterwards, his eye would become very dry. He suspected that the back treatment with his face down caused his eye problems. I said that I have not seen one single case of acupuncture causing extra tears, and I suggested that he see an ophthalmologist. In the mean time, he perspired a lot during the treatment. I explained to him that his alcohol intake produced a lot of internal heat, especially in his liver channel, which may be associated with his redness and the tearing in his left eye. I also told him that his tear ducts might be blocked for some reason. His eye check up showed inflammation of the left eye and drooping of the lower eyelid. His ophthalmologist suggested surgery to remove part of his eyelid.

I asked him to wait and allow me to treat him with acupuncture and herbs for a couple of months to see if we could relieve the symptoms before he jumped into surgery. He started once a week treatments in December. In the mean time, I was trying to convince him to cut down his red wine intake. His red eye went away after 4 treatments. At this point, he finally decided to stop the testosterone gel because his blood pressure was constantly high. With once a week acupuncture treatments, his sexual drive started to improve at the age of 55.

He still drank his glass of red wine every night with his meal. I noticed that his feet had poor circulation with constant sweating, coldness and hyper-sensitivity when I used alcohol to clean his feet. He argued that this is genetic because his dad also had the same hyper-reflex. I told him that it was associated with his alcohol intake. His tongue had many purple spots, and the sublingual vein looked enlarged and purple. Two months after acupuncture treatments for his eyes, his tearing was reduced and did not run down his face, but he still had to use antibiotic eye drops. Finally, he stopped drinking wine during the week because he was worried that his testosterone would go down again after he stopped his testosterone gel. We started Chinese herbal treatment. After three weeks, his eye pus decreased, so that he only needed to use antibiotic eye drops every three to four days. Furthermore, his sleep became much deeper after he stopped drinking alcohol. He also cut down sweets and coffee.

With only acupuncture once a week for 12 weeks, I was able to reduce his left eye tears so that they did not run down his face very often; his sleep became very deep, but pus came and went. I finally recommended that he continue take Chinese herbs for another month. He had tremendous blocked heat in his liver channel, and his circulation was not good, with many purple spots on his tongue and enlarged purple sublingual blood vessels. I tried to figure out why he had developed this eye condition. He used to be an amateur boxer and might have been hit in the left eye area, which could lead to lower eyelid drooping. Later, he found many cases on the Internet of men with drooping eyelids.

He had used Propecia, a prescribed medicine, to counteract the side effects of testosterone gel: hair loss, for six to nine months. This drug has been linked with the drooping of eyelids because it reduces muscle tone, including that of eyelid muscle. At this time, he finally cut down his alcohol intake to once a week in March 2008. After taking herbs for four months, his tear production became normal, with no pus coming out. He only occasionally needed to use his eye drops, the purple spots on his tongue disappeared, and the redness of his face was reduced. Furthermore, the hyper-reflex on his left foot went away, indicating a more balanced nervous system; he had not had a panic attack since he started acupuncture treatment.

During his yearly checkup for his kidney function, his urologist found out that his tiny tufts of capillaries, which carry blood within the kidneys, had a very low filtration rate; he was 55 years old, but the rate matched the kidney function of an 80-year-old man. My explanation was that dehydration due to his alcohol intake and not drinking enough water contributed to this kidney problem.

In this case, Mr. Rosenthal's daily stress, indigestion, intake of alcohol, sweets, and coffee, together with aging, led to his low testosterone, so that he started losing his libido and muscle mass. He automatically was given artificial testosterone, which caused accelerating hair loss. The next step, to save his hair, was Propecia, which caused his eyelid muscle drooping. Why did it happen to his left eye and not the right eye? Maybe it was an old injury from when he was boxing in his twenties.

He scheduled an eye operation in June 2008. Combining Chinese herbs and his weekly acupuncture treatment, however, enabled him to cancel the surgery and save the risk of this procedure and the time he would have lost.

His two cups of coffee in the morning increased his heartbeat and blood pressure dramatically. He cut down the coffee to one cup. After cutting down the alcohol intake, the purple spot on his tongue gradually disappeared. He was able to stop the antibiotic eye drops after six months of herbal intake. He gradually cut down alcohol intake to once a week. Interestingly, he started apple cider vinegar and found out that it helped to reduce the pus, but his sleep was reduced to 6 hours. When he stressed out, his left eye produced more pus. He also practiced Yoga twice a week. He was more refreshed in the morning after he stopped his daily wine intake.

The Science Behind My Treatment Methods for Mr. Rosenthal

Testosterone is a steroid hormone produced by the interstitial cells of the testes. The production of testosterone is controlled by a luteinizing hormone released from the anterior pituitary gland and is subject to a negative feedback mechanism. Therefore, if you have too much testosterone, the pituitary gland will reduce the amount of luteinizing hormone so that the testes produce less testosterone. On the other hand, if the testosterone level is too low, the pituitary will increase the amount of the stimulating hormone to push the testes to produce more testosterone.

The functions of testosterone

1. Testosterone is necessary for the proper development of the male reproductive system during puberty.

2. Following puberty, testosterone keeps the male reproductive system working properly, producing healthy sperm and seminal fluid.

3. Testosterone promotes sexual function and the sexual drive.

4. Testosterone initiates and maintains the secondary sex characteristics of males. Males exhibit increased muscular development, deepened voices, broad shoulders, prominent body and facial hair, and patterned baldness.

What can cause low testosterone levels and erectile dysfunction?

1. Stress: Research indicates that stress can lower testosterone levels temporarily, causing functional impotence. This effect is reversible, but if stress continues for too long, structural changes will also follow.

2. Medications: Certain medications, such as those that treat high blood pressure, anxiety, and depression (including the tricyclics and the monoamine oxidase inhibitors) have been implicated in erectile dysfunction, decreased libido, and impaired ejaculation. Calcium channel

blockers and acetylcholine esterase inhibitors cause a low incidence of erectile dysfunction. Although most high blood pressure medications have been associated with some kind of erectile impairment, diuretics seem to have little effect on erectile function. High blood pressure medications, which target the sympathetic nervous system, seldom cause impotence but may trigger retrograde ejaculation because they may relax the smooth muscles around the urethra and the bladder neck. Therefore, if one kind of blood pressure pill causes temporary impotence, you should try another kind.

Generally, erectile dysfunction due to drugs that contain selective serotonin reuptake inhibitors should resolve after discontinuing the medications. However, in the 2008 issue of the *Journal of Sex Medicine*, Dr. Csoka et al. at the University of Pittsburgh reported three cases in which sexual dysfunctions such as low libido, the inability to achieve orgasm, the loss of sensation in the genital area, and erectile dysfunction did not return to normal after the patients stopped taking selective serotonin reuptake inhibitors (SSRIs).

What to tell Your Chinese Medicine Doctor

To reduce the stress and restore the normal level of testosterone:

Herbal formula: Chai Hu 12g, Chi Shao 15g, Zhi Qiao 15g, Ba Ji Tian 12g, Shan Yao 15g, Huai Niu Xi 15g, Tu Si Zi 12g, Gou Qi Zi 12g, Mei Gui Hua 6g, Dang Gui 12g

Points for improving the testicular and pituitary functions:

1. CV2 (Qiu Gu): at the midpoint of the upper border of the symphysis pubis.

2. CV4 (Guan Yuan): On the anterior median line of the lower abdomen, 3 cun below the bellybutton.

3. GV4 (Ming Men): on the posterior median line of the back, in the depression below the spinous process of the 2nd lumbar vertebra.

4. UB23 (Shen Shu): On the back, 1.5 cun lateral to the lower border of the spinous process of the 2nd lumbar vertebra.

5. Kid12 (Da He): On the lower abdomen, 4 cun below the center of the bellybutton, .5 cun lateral to the anterior midline.

6. Kid2 (Ran Gu): On the medial aspect of the foot, below the tuberosity of the navicular bone, at the junction of the red and white skin.

Chapter 11

Vertigo

V ertigo, an American psychological film, was directed by Alfred Hitchcock and starred James Stewart and Kim Novak. In the film, a retired police detective who suffers from acrophobia was hired as a private investigator to follow the wife of an acquaintance and uncover the mystery of her peculiar behavior. This movie is now frequently ranked among the greatest films ever made. In this movie, the courses of people's lives are changed forever because of this illness. In the clinical case that follows, you'll see close-up the impact on a real life and the steps to release from this physically and psychologically damaging ailment.

A woman walked into my office on unsteady feet. Judith Malady is a distinguished and beautiful woman, who has been married happily for 30 years and has had vertigo since her early childhood. She came to me in a state of distress because vertigo was making her dizzy even when she just simply turned her head. How many times do we do that in a day, I thought?

Vertigo had been a problem since her youth. In high school, when her new boyfriend asked her to go to the county fair on her first date, she had to refuse for fear that he would suspect her illness when she refused to go on any of the rides, since certainly a roller coaster would set her off. Even riding in a car could make her dizzy. I was surprised to hear, however, that, if she rode in a car with other people, she tended to feel dizzy, but if *she* were driving, she would not feel so bad. Therefore, I started to question her daily living habits. I found out many things. My private investigator side came out to see if it could solve this case. I found out that if she ate greasy and salty food, the dizziness would be worse when she rode in a car. It is understood in Chinese medicine that the indigestion of greasy food will cause the body to produce phlegm or abnormal water retention, which in some people can cause dizziness. In the past, when I treated such a condition, I tried to improve digestion first.

Ms. Malady had been a successful business woman at the age of forty. She became the CEO of a biotech company in the Boston area. Her life became so busy that she could only sleep 5 to 6 hours most of the time. She had to drink a lot of coffee, sometimes 5 or 6 cups to get her going in the morning. Surprisingly, the caffeine never made her irritable. I found out through the grapevine that people in her company found her easy to work with and an inspirational boss. People who drive themselves this hard often have excessive adrenalin release, which initiates the "fight or flight" type responses to interactions, but not Judith. However, with such a constant adrenaline release, sometimes people miss body alerts that say, "please take care of this problem." One time she sprained her ankle without knowing it. She came in to see me one day for acupuncture, and I said "Judith, what caused your swollen ankle?" She looked at me quizzically, and said, "what swollen ankle?" Wow, can you believe it? This is a common occurrence for such people.

Additionally, she had developed seasonal allergies with sneezing, tearing and having itchy eyes since her childhood. She was noticing that her vertigo became worse whenever her stress increased. Coincidentally, her allergic symptoms got worse as well. During seasonal allergies, her histamine level may go up, and this may lead to dizziness. That is why physicians use anti-histamines to treat vertigo. The other three hormones involved in dizziness are dopamine, norepinephrine, and acetylcholine. When these three chemical levels increase abnormally, you may feel dizzy. Stress can increase our dopamine and norepinephrine levels, thus inducing vertigo. On the other hand, GABA can reduce vertigo by inhibiting the neurons involved in dizziness.

I continued to treat Judith. We had been working together for some time, and all her physical check-ups had been normal, including her liver function. By stopping her coffee, cutting down salt and simple sugar, her vertigo only erupted with her allergies when seasons changed or when she became dehydrated. The vertigo could reappear occasionally when she quickly turned to the right side, but she had no vertigo when getting up from lying down or sitting, when driving, skiing or hiking. The sensor for this head movement is very sensitive in Judith, which may be associated with long-term seasonal allergies and genetic factors. Interestingly, she had been practicing yoga for many years, although certain yoga positions always triggered her vertigo. She finally decided to give up yoga, and instead she only does certain stretching exercises now. After a year of once-a-week acupuncture treatment, her vertigo is almost gone.

What Caused Vertigo in Judith Malady.

In most people, vertigo is caused by a problem of the inner ear. Inside your ear there is a tiny organ called the vestibular labyrinth. It includes loop-shaped structures (semicircular canals) that contain fluid and fine, hair-like sensors that monitor the rotation of your head. Other structures (otolith organs) in your ear monitor linear movements of your head and your head's position relative to gravity. These otolith organs contain crystals that make you sensitive to movement. For a variety of reasons, some of these crystals can become dislodged and move into one of the semicircular canals — especially while you're lying down. This causes the semicircular canal to become sensitive to head positional changes it would normally not respond to. As a result, you feel dizzy. The sensation of movement or imbalance when you are not moving is called vertigo, and vertigo when you change your head position is called benign positional vertigo. In Judith's case, genetically her sensor for head movement is very sensitive, which explains why she never enjoys riding roller coasters. When she was young, her heavy drinking of coffee as an Italian, lack of water intake and work stress put her immune function out of balance, so that she developed seasonal allergies. With high histamine and norepinephirne levels during her episodes of allergy, the little sensor in her inner ear became super sensitive.

What Causes Vertigo?

Viral infection

Inner ear surgery

Head injury

Too much aspirin, Phenytoin and/or alcohol

Nerve inflammation

Severe cold exposure

Dehydration

Prolonged lying on the back

Bell's Palsy

What are the Symptoms of Vertigo?

Dizziness: A sense that you or your surroundings are spinning or moving (vertigo), lightheadedness

Unsteadiness

Loss of balance

Blurred vision associated with the sensation of vertigo

Nausea

Vomiting

Abnormal rhythmic eye movements (pathological nystagmus)

What can You Do to Heal Yourself?

1. The positional exercises of Brandt and Daroff: Sit on the edge of the bed near the middle, with legs hanging down. Turn head 45° to right side. Quickly lie down on left side, with head still turned, and touch the bed with the portion of the head behind the ear. Maintain this position and every subsequent position for about thirty seconds. Stand up again for thirty seconds. Quickly lie down to right side after turning

head 45° toward the left side. Stand up again. Do 6-10 repetitions, 3 times per day. These exercises may desensitize certain sensors in your inner ear.

2. Drink a lot of water to avoid dehydration. When you are dehydrated, you have insufficient blood flow to your head, so that your blood pressure fluctuates too much when you change position. Also, dehydration can induce histamine release. Here is a case to explain how important water is to your health. An 80-year-old, very healthy, man came to my clinic. He had been very healthy and still played tennis two hours every day. He suddenly developed vertigo and went through all the medical tests without any positive findings. When he came to see me, I did a physical exam and found out that his neck was very stiff. I asked him if he drank a lot of water. He said to me that he drank some, not too convincingly. I suggested that he stretch his neck muscles and drink plenty of water. Since he played tennis for two to four hours every day, he might be dehydrated chronically if nobody reminded him to drink water, which happens a lot with men that I have treated for some reasons. These two factors contributed to his lack of blood flow to his inner ear and dysfunction of the vestibular labyrinth (the sensor for head positional changes).

3. Have your allergies treated: When you have allergies, your sensor for head position can function abnormally due to swelling or

inflammation. You can drink one teaspoon of apple cider vinegar 3 times a day to improve your digestion and reduce your allergies.

4. Get plenty of rest to rejuvenate your adrenal gland in order to reduce the inflammation of the inner ear. The adrenal gland produces cortisol to fight inflammation and allergy and maintain blood pressure and blood sugar level.

5. Balance your hormones: Estrogen and progesterone imbalance can cause vertigo. One of my patients had vertigo for a long time. When going to sleep, she would lie on her stomach or lie on her back without a pillow, because her positional sensor was too sensitive otherwise. When she got pregnant, her dizziness got worse. The hormone changes sensitized the nerves in her inner ear. Also, high progesterone during pregnancy may have caused swelling in her inner ear. When her allergies got worse, her dizziness also got worse due to increased histamine levels. If, after not having dizziness, she did not sleep well for a couple of nights or became overly stressed for a period of time, her dizziness came back. Insufficient sleep may cause imbalance of the nervous system, and a low cortisol level can also cause dysfunction of the nerves.

Bring This to Your Traditional Chinese Medicine Doctor

Acupuncture points

GB12: posterior to the ear, in the depression posterior and inferior to the mastoid process.

GB10: On the head, posterior to the ear, posterior and superior to the mastoid process, at the junction of the middle 1/3 and upper 1/3 of the arc connecting GB 9 and GB 12.

GB41: On the lateral side of the dorsum of the foot, proximal to the 4th metatarsophalangeal joint, between the 4th and 5th metatarsal bones, on the lateral side of the tendon of m. extensor digiti minimi of the foot.

Chinese Herbal Treatment:

1. Phlegm condition:

Symptoms: dizziness when head turns to a certain position, overweight, tendency to have cysts or lipomas, nasal congestion, post-nasal drip, feeling heavy when humidity increases, cloudy head, still feeling tired after sleeping more than 8 hours. Tongue: pale or purple with white greasy coating, Pulse: soggy or slippery.

Herbal formula: Ban Xia 6g, Bai Zhu 10g, Ze Xie 10g, Tian Ma 10g, Shi Chang Pu 10g, Fu Ling 15g, Chuan Bei Mu 6g. If there are heat symptoms: add Zhu Ru 6g, Dan Nan Xing 6g.

2. Liver Yang Rising with kidney Yin deficiency:

Symptoms: Dizziness that gets worse when you get angry or stressed out, neck stiffness, red face with high blood pressure, dry skin, always thirsty, hair loss, premature ejaculation, low back pain, warm sensation in palms or bottoms of the feet, hot flushes with night sweats sometimes, constipation. Tongue: bright red with little coating or dry white coating, pulse: thin and fast.

Herbal formula: Bai Shao 12g, Gui Ban 15g, Xuan Shen 12g, Dai Zhe Shi 15g, Long Gu 20g, Mu Li 15g, Chao Mai Ya 15g, Chuan Niu Xi 12g, Chuan Lian Zi 6g, Tian Men Dong 12g, Zhi Gan Cao 6g.

3. Liver and heart fire interrupts orifice.

Symptoms: Tendency to over think, waking up early in the morning with compulsive thinking about one specific thing, red eyes, blood pressure either high or low, very thin constitution, irritability. Chinese Herbal Formula:

Herbal formula: Buffalo Horn 20g, Gou Teng 15g, Fu Shen 20g, Hang Ju Hua 6g, Chi shao 12g, Sheng Di 12g, Huang Lian 3g, Dan Zhu Ye 12g, Mu Dan Pi 9g, Zhi Zi 6g.

Chapter Twelve

Cancer

Writing this chapter makes me happy. Why, you say, would writing about cancer elicit happiness in anyone? Well, I'll tell you. I practiced Chinese Medicine alongside oncologists at the Dana Farber Cancer Institute, a teaching hospital of the Harvard Medical School, located in Boston. I admit that watching more and more people being diagnosed with cancer motivates me to write this chapter, in hopes of helping people avoid this disease or have a faster recovery from it.

I imagine that you are surprised to see a chapter dedicated to cancer in a book about Chinese Medicine. The truth is that much of my practice supports the treatment of all types of cancer. It is a very serious, deadly disease. I would never tell you to only employ Chinese Medicine in treating this killer, but I will tell you that Chinese Medicine is used both as a preventative protocol and a very important adjunct to a full treatment regimen for many types of cancers.

There are no typical cases of cancer. The case study that I present to you is one of which I have detailed knowledge. This man has been an important member of the community, an acquaintance of my family, as well as a patient. I have changed his name to protect his privacy.

I have known David Lin, a Chinese scientist, for much of my life. His mother died of lung cancer at the age of 83, without any chemotherapy or radiation therapy, while his father died of pancreatic cancer at the age of 82. As a child, he was healthy and full of energy. He would ice skate, play football or swim in a small pond for a whole day, and then come home to eat, so it was a shock to me when he developed cancer at the age of 73. His mother had been so busy taking care of his big family that she did not have time to remind him to drink water or eat his vegetables and fruits, but he loved to eat apples and peanuts and would often eat five apples at one time. I guess the fruit helped to make up some of the water his body really needed. He never drank alcohol or smoked. His blood pressure and heart rate had been very low.

He had been one of the smartest boys in his hometown in the Northeastern part of China. By his own effort and hard work, he was admitted to the most prestigious university in China. He then wrote 5 books and published more than one hundred scientific papers.

He was an active man. He rode his bike to work every day. He had a well-rounded diet, without all the sweets available today. In China before the 1970s, candy and other desserts were really not available. Every family was allocated only 1.7 pounds of sugar every month. However, because he was chronically dehydrated, he had two problems since his college study: one was a chronic infection in his nose and throat. The other was severe migraines. His repetitive upper respiratory infection led to chronic inflammation and later polyps inside his nose. At the age of 28, his polyps were surgically removed without anesthesia. The pain was beyond a normal person's tolerance. Dr. Lin had been a tough man, but after this surgery, he desperately walked in the city of Beijing for a whole day to calm himself down. The traumatic pain left a major impact in his brain, and he avoided any kind of surgical procedure afterwards. He had migraines, which I think was associated with his chronic water and vitamin deficiency that caused an abnormal functioning of his blood vessels.

At 50 years old, his financial condition greatly improved due to his academic achievements, and this changed his eating habits. He would buy a bag of cookies and eat it before dinner. At dinnertime, he ate hardly any vegetables. This pattern lasted for 15 years. Gradually, in his early sixties, he started to experience health problems. He began to lose sleep due to severe knee pain. The knee pain did not bother his daily activities, but at night the pain was so severe that he had to kneel down on his bed until 2 AM. Because he was thereby sleep deprived, stress hormones would increase significantly the next day. Eventually he depleted his adrenal gland. His blood pressure had been very low, so his blood circulation was compromised.

He worked hard until he was 65 years of age, when he retired and came to America to take care of his grandchildren. He developed glaucoma at the age of 68. Initially the ophthalmologist tried to use eye drops to lower his eye pressure. Even with quite low eye pressure (11 to 12), his visual field continued to be damaged. His acupuncturist observed his eye pressure for two years and found no relationship between his eye pressure and visual field damage. In the meantime, he used eye drops twice a day. These were very strong, and his eyes burned so badly that he could hardly read for more than 10 minutes on any given day. His ophthalmologist claimed that it was a tradeoff between this dry and burning sensation and low eye pressure. He continued acupuncture treatment to improve eye blood circulation, then he started cutting down his eye drops to once a day.

After two months, surprisingly, his eye pressure stayed quite low, and his visual field stopped changing. This implied that the poor blood circulation had been causing his visual field damage and eye pressure increase. Acupuncture facilitated blood circulation to the eye area. That is why he always said that his vision became instantly better right after each of his acupuncture treatments.

After Dr. Lin's retirement, he also increased his water intake, and his migraines did not come back for more than 8 years. However, it was very hard to change his life-long eating habits: not enough vegetables and fruits. Due to his lack of sleep and vitamin deficit, his nervous system started changing. He was never afraid of anything before he reached his sixties. He led visiting scholars to many countries including Germany, Turkey, Japan and the USA. Now he developed claustrophobia and depression, so that he could not even take the subway or fly in an airplane because of irrational fears. He would suddenly develop anxiety if his patient name bracelets were too tight or if the airplane or train did not move for a while. I guess his sympathetic nerves may have become too sensitive due to a deficiency of vitamins and serotonin. The lowered serotonin level also caused a chronic deficiency of melatonin. He could only sleep 3 to 4 hours per night now, even though he had been a good sleeper until he reached his 60s. The other sign of a super-sensitive nervous system was a tendency for his legs to vibrate if there was any stimulation on his foot or legs, including acupuncture needles.

Since he stopped working at the age of 65, he had been unhappy, and his insomnia had become worse. He developed a chronic cough in the winter, probably due to eating extremely salty dry nuts or too many sweets. His voice was constantly hoarse. He should have had an x-ray done, but his fear of hospitals persisted. Every time he started coughing during the winter, his daughter would ask him to drink more water. His cough gradually went away, but chronic inflammation remained for years. Last winter, while visiting his son in New Jersey, he had been eating milk chocolate, cookies and other sweets every day. After only two-and-a-half months, he developed persistent coughing and difficulty breathing. He was diagnosed with advanced lung cancer due to repetitive infection and imbalanced immune function. Since he is Asian and a non-smoker, his oncologist started a protocol of Tarsevar to shrink his tumor. He developed rashes, mouth sores and other symptoms. One day, after he took his medication in the morning on an empty stomach, his lung water suddenly increased, and his heart also became surrounded by water. This happened because Tarsevar not only attacks cancer cells but can also damage lung and pericardial lining cells. His healthy heart then began working so hard to maintain oxygen levels that he could have developed heart failure if not admitted to the hospital right away. The thoracic surgeon dug three holes in his chest to drain out the fluid from his pericardium and lungs. He was carrying seven tubes and was given a high dosage painkiller every 6 hours. Since he never smoked or drank alcohol, his heart and lung function was strong. After surgery, the next day, he started walking with seven tubes connected to different containers. Three days later, Dr. Lin left the hospital, determined to conquer his cancer. He was so weak that his body could not afford another type of chemotherapy right after surgery.

His acupuncturist and herbalist did acupuncture every other day to rebuild his vital energy, asking him to eat brown rice porridge and five-element soup religiously. He was so scared of being hospitalized again that he started eating more vegetables and completely stopped eating sweets. His granddaughter cooked his raw herbs every other day, the brown rice porridge and five-element soup twice a week. Every morning when he woke up, he drank his five-element soup to clean out the toxin from chemotherapy. Then he would eat his anti-cancer brown rice porridge, followed by herbs once in the morning and once in the afternoon. After three-and-a-half months, his 5x3 inch cancer mass was dramatically reduced, and there was no water accumulating in his right lung. Furthermore, his bone metastasis on his thoracic vertebra had become stenosed, meaning the cancer cells were not active any more in that part of the bone. He was not as strong as he was 10 years earlier, but, with some care, he should be able to live a relatively healthy life for the next several years.

From this case, we can reach the following conclusion: if you are lucky enough to live in a safe, non-toxic environment in your childhood and can eat healthy foods until you are in your fifties, your body can adjust itself until you reach sixty years of age, even though you do not want to drink water and do not eat enough fruits and vegetables. After that, your aging process starts to speed up. You might develop cancer, arthritis or an autoimmune disease. The earlier you spend time and money to take care of your body, the better quality of life you will have. On the other hand, if a child starts eating junk after he reaches 1 year old, by the age of forty, most of his blood vessels and nerves will be inflamed. Furthermore, if he does not have good sleep, with a high-stress job and a deficiency of vitamins, his chromosomes are very likely to mutate by the age of forty. It would be difficult to get a 10-year survival rate from chemotherapy treatment because cancer cell growth is relatively fast in a forty-year-old man, compared to a seventy-year-old man. This sounds very harsh, I know. Growing old is not for the faint of heart.

Cancer is part of the aging process. Almost everyone has some cancer cells in his or her body. As long as we have a strong immune system, the cancer cells are well under control, so take good care of yourself by combining Western and Chinese medicine. It's the best chance we have.

The Science behind My Treatment Methods for Dr. David Lin

What can contribute to the development of cancer? Cancer is the abnormal growth of immature cells in an uncontrollable way and can spread to other parts of the body. Cancer starts when our chromosomes are damaged by oxidation, radiation, stress, or an imbalance of hormones and the nervous system.

Over time I have developed a list of direct and indirect causes or conditions that can lead to cancer, based on extensive research. If you would like to view these research studies, which I reference, please review my well-documented medical research book entitled "Acupuncture and Hormone Balance" available at Lulu.com. Here's the Cliff Notes version of factors that can contribute to cancer development:

1. Chronic inflammation in certain body areas such as intestine and prostate.

2. Hormone imbalance: imbalance of estrogen and progesterone leads to overgrowth of breast tissue, uterus lining or ovarian tissues. This growth is usually benign, but it can become cancerous under certain conditions.

3. Stress can cause an imbalance of immune function, thus weakening it.

4. Too much ultraviolet light can damage the skin, causing melanoma.

5. Cigarette smoking.

6. Too much junk food is linked with chronic inflammation.

7. Lack of sleep can lead to weakened immune function and imbalance of hormones.

8. Deficiency of Vitamin D due to indigestion and lack of sunshine exposure.

Why are more and more young people developing cancer in this society?

Too much sugar can cause chronic inflammation, leading to mutation of chromosomes.

Sleeping at the wrong time or lack of sleep can cause imbalance of immune function.

Chemotherapy, radiation therapy and surgery are very good treatments to remove or control tumors very quickly, but these treatments can potentially damage your liver, kidney, immune and digestive systems. The following self-healing techniques will help you to achieve the highest survival rate if properly combined with the surgery, chemotherapy and radiation therapy.

Self-healing techniques:

Five-element vegetable soup: daikon 200 g, daikon leaves 200 g, dried mushroom 200 g, carrots 200 g and Niu Bang (Burdock) 200 g; add 1200 cc water and boil the vegetables for an hour. You can buy all these ingredients from the Whole Food market.

You can drink this soup (250-500 cc) every day to improve your digestive system and maintain your blood count 72 hours after your chemotherapy. This soup also can help your liver to clean out the toxins after the chemotherapy treatment. Many advanced cancer patients have a very good response to chemotherapy initially, but they do not protect their digestive function. Instead they eat a lot of sweet stuff to make themselves happy temporarily. In Chinese medicine, it is thought that the sweets can cause bloating and nausea when you try to eat vegetables and whole grains. Your stomach cannot absorb the valuable nutrients from whole foods. Eventually, anemia is so bad that you cannot tolerate chemotherapy because of the deficiency of nutrients. The immune function declines to the point that it does not protect you anymore, and by that time the cancer has started to spread.

Develop good eating habits in early stages of chemotherapy, while your digestive function is still normal. Try to eat more vegetables and fruits because the anti-oxidants of natural fruits will help your body fight cancer. If you really crave sweets, reward yourself a little bit after your finish your main meal or just substitute the sweets with fruits. We need to create an alkali internal condition so that cancer cells cannot survive.

Brown rice Porridge: water 1000 1500 ml, brown rice 0.75 cup, lotus 0.5 lb (peeled and cut into cubes), large-rooted mustard (Asian kohlrabi) 0.4 lb, Tremella fuciformis fungus (Bai Mu Er) 1 cup (remove the hard parts and soak in water until soft). Boil the water, add the above ingredients, and let it sit for about half an hour. Then add the following ingredients: cauliflower 0.5 lb, carrots 0.5 lb (peeled and sliced and stir fried in olive oil first), cabbage 0.5 lb, yam 0.5 lb (peeled and cut into cubes), and walnuts 1/2 cup.

Cook everything for another half hour. Cool down the porridge, pour it into a glass jar, and store in the refrigerator. This formula was invented by a Chinese nutritionist, Ms. He (San Diego, California). Cancer patients should take this soup while they are having chemotherapy. Ms. He has many success stories about advanced cancer patients who lived up to more than 10 years, whereas conventional medicine only gave them a couple of months to live.

Anti-cancer soup 1: brown rice 300g, asparagus 300g, tropical mushroom 300g, Yi Yi Ren 300g, water 500cc. Add a small amount of sea salt and cook for an hour. Eat a small bowl of this soup every morning.

Anti-cancer soup 2: sea weed 200g, Fig (Wu Hua guo) 200g, organic shellfish 300g, water 500 cc, one organic egg white; boil the above ingredients for 15 minutes.

Anti-cancer soup 3: Auricularia auricula (Hei Mu Er) 200g, corn 20 g, Reishi (Ling Zhi) 200g, water 500cc, boiled for 25 min.

Avoid toasted, baked and deep fried meat. Protein is not easily digested if cooked in these ways. Furthermore, when meat is heated above 100^0C, it tends to produce carcinogenic chemicals. Boiled or steamed meat is the best source of our protein. We can add basil or sage leaves to make it tasty.

Have only a small amount of spicy food once a week, because spicy food creates a lot of internal heat, which can potentially cause inflammation inside your body.

Stop drinking alcohol if you are diagnosed with cancer, as it can cause more imbalances in your system. Alcohol can damage your liver, your nerves and your blood vessels.

Avoid greasy foods, which are hard to digest and can upset your digestive system. Your nausea, vomiting, queasy stomach, mouth sores and diarrhea or constipation will get worse if the food cannot be digested properly. During chemotherapy, the stomach and intestinal membranes are inflamed, so you need to eat easily digested food, such as soup.

Practice Qigong and Tai Chi to smooth your energy flow. Choose an area where there is not much traffic and that has many pine trees, so when you take deep breaths, you get fresh air to nourish your whole body.

Drink 8 cups of water to cleanse your kidneys, as you need to urinate at least every two hours right after your chemotherapy.

Avoid eating red meat with hormones and antibiotics. The hormones can stimulate the cancer to grow even faster.

If you have breast cancer, you have to cut down strong coffee intake, because it will stimulate insulin release and insulin as a growth factor could stimulate the tissue growth. Research shows that high insulin levels are associated with lower survival rates from prostate and breast cancer.

Avoid simple sugars to maintain a healthy insulin level. Please remember that high insulin levels can lead to inflammation. If you love chocolate, cookies, cakes, and ice cream, please cut down to once a week or even to every other week after you finish all your healthy food. You only feel good for one hour when you eat that kind of stuff.

Be happy all the time. There is nothing more important than your health. When you are happy, your immune function will be strengthened. That is why some cancer survivors can heal themselves. One of my dad's friends was diagnosed with lung cancer. He finished all the treatments in Beijing, and then he went to a rural area where the air is fresh. He and his wife became very serious gardeners, and he has been cancer free for many years.

Acupuncture helps to improve digestion, immune function, and adrenal gland function and reduce your stress level. Most cancer centers integrate acupuncture as an adjunct treatment to chemotherapy or radiation therapy. According to Dr. Sencer of Children's Hospital of Minneapolis, acupuncture has become part of conventional treatments in many American Hospitals, just as in China. During chemotherapy or radiation therapy, I recommend to have acupuncture twice a week. After you finish the chemotherapy, change to once a week for 3 months, then every other week for another three months, then once a month for a year. If you maintain a healthy life style, you may have acupuncture when the season changes, which will help your body restore its balance.

Get enough sleep by practicing relaxation techniques, such as stretching, Yoga, or Qi Gong 2 hours before you go to bed. You need at least 6 to 8 hours of non-interrupted sleep to rejuvenate your immune function. You have to go to bed before 12PM. According to Chinese medicine, the energy flow to each individual internal organ happens at a certain time. For instance, from 11 PM to 1 AM, the gallbladder starts secretion and discharges toxins from the body. Also, bone marrow produces new blood cells. From 1 to 3 AM, your cells are repairing. The liver discharges toxins, and your body produces a lot of hormones and antibodies. From 3 to 5 AM, the cortisol level is the lowest, and there is less blood flow to the brain. Bone marrow finishes its job. Very sick people tend to die during this time. We need to relax, digest and repair between 10 PM to 6 AM. If you have a party until 2 or 3 AM, your body will miss the time to repair itself. Sleep during the daytime is not the same as during the night because the repair work is more efficient during the night. That is Mother Nature's cycle.

After chemotherapy, if a patient has dry mouth and coughing, use this medicinal tea: Bi Qi (Chinese Bayberry) 200 g, snow pear 200 g, fresh Tuber Ophiopogonis Japonici (Mai Dong) 200 g, fresh lotus 200 g, fresh Phregmites (Lu gen) 200 g, cane sugar 50 g, water 1000 cc. Cook with low grade fire for 20 minutes. Drink it as a tea. If you do not need cane sugar to adjust the taste, it is better not to add it.

Lung Cancer patients: Ji Cai (Capsella bursa-pastoris) 200 g, Yi Yi Ren 200 g, add water 500 cc and cook for half an hour; eat this porridge once or twice a day to strengthen your digestive function and expel the pathological water.

To relieve dry coughing, anemia and fatigue: cook brown rice 400 g with Bai He (Bulbus Lilili) 200 g, Wild Tremella (Yin Er) 100 g and red bean 400 g, for an hour. Eat one cup of soup once a day.

To restore the liver function and raise the blood count: cook organic chicken with Wu Wei Zi (Schizandrae) 200 g and drink the chicken soup.

Steam duck with *Ginkgo biloba* L. (Yin Xing) to relieve the dry cough.

Lung Cancer:

More people have this type of cancer than any other, both men and women. Evidence-based guidelines published by the American College of Chest Physicians in September 2007 recommends acupuncture for lung cancer patients experiencing fatigue, difficulty to breath, chemotherapy-induced neuropathy, or to soothe symptoms of pain, nausea and vomiting.

Acupuncture points:

Relieve coughing and breathing difficulty:

Tian Tu (CV22): On the anterior median line of the neck, in the center of the suprasternal fossa.

Xuan Ji (CV21): On the anterior median line of the chest, 1.0 cun below Tian Tu.

Tan Zhong (CV17): On the anterior median line of the chest, at the level of the 4th intercostal space, at the midpoint between the two nipples.

Chi Ze (Lu5): On the cubital crease, on the radial side of the tendon m. biceps brachii.

Fei Shu (UB13): On the back, 1.5 cun lateral to the lower border of the spinous process of the 3rd thoracic vertebra.

Pi Shu (UB21): On the back, 1.5 cun lateral to the lower border of the spinous process of the 11th thoracic vertebra.

Guan Yuan Shu (UB26): On the back, 1.5 cun lateral to the lower border of the spinous process of the 5th lumbar vertebra.

Tai Yuan (Lu9): On the radial end of the transverse crease of the wrist, where the radial artery pulsates.

If wheezing is the main symptom:

Jing Qiu (Lu8): on the radial palmar aspect of the forearm, in the depression between the styloid process of the radius and the radial artery, 1 cun above the transverse crease of the wrist.

If you have diarrhea from chemotherapy, then the following:

Shou San Li (LI10): with the elbow flexed, the point is on the dorsal radial side of the forearm, on the line connecting LI 5 and LI 11, 2 cun below the transverse cubital crease.

Headache with chemo drug:

He Gu (LI4): between the 1st and 2nd metacarpal bones, in the middle of the 2nd metacarpal bone on the radial side.

Bai Hui (GV20): at the midpoint of the line connecting the apexes of the two auricles.

Coughing with anxiety, insomnia and palpitation:

Shen Tang (UB44): on the back, 3.0 cun lateral to the lower border of the spinous process of the 5th thoracic vertebra.

Hua Gai (CV20): On the anterior median line of the chest, at the level of the 1st intercostal space.

Chinese Herbal Formula based on differentiated Patterns:

1. Wind with phlegm in upper burner: itchy throat, dry cough, few phlegm or phlegm with foams, chest tightness, Tongue: light red, thin white coating, Pulse: floating.

Treatment Principle: expel wind, transform the phlegm and open lung qi to stop coughing

Herbal formula: Zi Su Ye 10g, Zi Su Zi 10g, Jie Geng 10g, Sheng Gan Cao 10g, Niu Bang Zi 6g, Qian Hu 6g, Xing Ren 10g, Quan Gua Lou 20g, Lu Gen 20g, Ban Xia 10g, Ban Zhi Lian 6g, Bai Hua She She Cao 6g.

If patient is currently having chemotherapy, do not add any Ban Zhi Lian and Bai Hua She She Cao.

2. Dampness and phlegm in middle and upper burner with heat:

Symptoms: coughing, chest tightness, cloudy head, decreased appetite, thirsty but does not want to drink, nausea, and vomiting, constipation, irritability.

Tongue: red with yellow thick greasy coating. Pulse: slippery.

Herbal formula: Fa Ban Xia 12g, Chen Pi 9g, Fu Ling 15g, Sheng Gan Cao 6g, Xing Ren 10g, Sha Ren 6g Zhi Shi 6g, Quan Gua Lou 10g, Huang Qin 10g, Dan Nan Xing 6g, Chao Mai Ya 20g.

3. Coughing with a lot of phlegm, wheezing and irritability:

Herbal formula: Fu Hai Shi 12g, Su Zi 12g, Bai Jie Zi 12g, Jie Geng 6g, Dan Zhu Ye 12g, Lian qiao 6g, Huang Qin 6g, Zhi Shi 6g, Dan Nan Xing 6g.

4. If fluids have accumulated in lower legs and lungs:

Herbal formula: Ze Xie 20g, Sheng Bai Zhu 10g, Fu ling 15g, Zhu Ling 10g, Ting Li Zi 10g, Gui Zhi 6g, Sheng Huang Qi 10g, Hong Zao 5g.

5. After surgery and chemotherapy, qi and Yin deficiency: fatigue, dry mouth, insomnia, light headed and decreased appetite.

Strengthen the spleen and lung, tonify the Yin and Qi.

Herbal formula: Huang Qi 20g, Sha Shen 15g, Tai Zi Shen 15g, Mai Dong 10g, Xing Ren 10g, Cang Zhu 6g, Ho Pu 6g, Zhe Bei Mu 6g, Chen Pi 6g, Yuan Zhi 10g, Fu Ling 15g. Xi Yang Shen 15g.

6. If left lung and kidney pulses are very weak, but both Guan pulses are slippery, lung and kidney deficiency and excess phlegm heat in the middle burner exist at the same time:

Add Zhe Bei Mu 10g, Chao Bai Zhu 15g, Xi Yang Shen 20g, Yi Yi Ren 20g, Ba Ji Tian 10g, Zhi Zi 6g.

Food Therapy for lung cancer:

If coughing blood:

Cook Jing Mi 100g, Da Zao 5g in 0.5 gallon water for 30 min; add Bai Ji15g, San Qi powder5g and honey two tea spoons at the end, drink 5 oz three times a day.

Cook Gan Cao 10g, snow pear 200 g, pig lung 250g. cut pear into cubes, wash pig lung and squeeze out the foam, slice it; add a small amount of Chinese rock sugar (Bing Tang), add some water to cover everything, cook for 2 hours, drink the soup 200 cc once a day.

Boost immune and digestive function after chemo or radiation therapy:

Gou Qi Zi 30g, Shan Yao 30g, Huang Qin 10g in 500 cc water, cooked for 20 min. Drink 100 cc twice a day.

217

Chapter 13

Migraine Headache

A 53-year-old business woman had suffered with migraine headaches since she was 13 years old. Her last period occurred at the age of 52. Her menopause symptoms were not bad. Patient did not use any hormones. However, 3 years before her last period, her migraines became more frequent and intense. Patient started taking Amitriptyline more often to relieve the debilitating migraines. Initially, after she took this magic pill, her migraine went away within a few hours, but she was exhausted and could hardly function. Therefore, she always delayed until the last minute to take this pill. Patient tried to cut down on her chocolate, wine and other possible triggers.

Interestingly, patient had a root canal two years ago. Since then, every time she had migraine, her toothache started. She noticed that all her problems were on her right side: right side migraine, back pain, varicose veins, breast cysts and ovarian cyst. One of the reasons is that she overused her right side, which became the weaker side. When there are imbalances, the right side cannot compensate anymore, all the symptoms show up on her right side.

When patient first came to see me, she was having migraines every day. Patient is a very motivated businesswoman with four children. Patient does not drink coffee, is weight appropriate, and drinks red wine only once a week. Despite patient following a generally healthy diet, she was having some indigestion problems: bloating, gas and constipation. Together we revisited all her habits and diets. I discovered that she was drinking 3 to 5 cups of tea per day. With this much tea, her digestion would slow down, so that vitamins and minerals could not be absorbed efficiently. Without sufficient vitamins and minerals, her nerves would become very sensitive to environmental changes: cold, heat, and humidity. After menopause, it is natural for our digestive and nervous systems to become very unstable, and we get stressed out easily. If we eat a little bit too much or too late, our blood sugar will go up too high or drop too low, and we may end up with indigestion and migraine. Plus, patient had ovarian cysts, varicose veins, and breast cysts, indicating that her estrogen was not balanced with progesterone before menopause. After menopause, the imbalance would become worse, with about a 70% decline in progesterone and 50% decline of estrogen. That is one of the reasons her migraines had become even worse.

I recommended that patient was to drink only one to two bags of tea every day and drink more water instead. Patient had noticed that if she were dehydrated, her migraine started. On one occasion, after she drank a lot of wine without enough water, her migraine became so bad that even her magic pills could not stop it. She was rushed to an emergency room to get a morphine drip; patient was unable to attend to her business that day.

Patient had also noticed that if she became too busy and forgot to eat lunch or drink enough water, she might get severe migraines on the next day. Patient was aware that chocolate could trigger the migraines. After patient reduced chocolate consumption, drank more water, and cut down her tea intake, her sleep got deeper. With only two acupuncture treatments, the frequency of her migraines decreased to every other week.

Her migraines occurred around her right eye and temple area. Patient said that when she applied pressure on the right side of her neck or head, the migraine pain decreased indicating that neck muscle tightness was aggravating her migraine. After another two acupuncture treatments, patient only gets migraines once every 7 weeks.

On one occasion, after the patient went out for a meal of pizza with diet coke in a restaurant, the salty food and sugar substitute induced a migraine the next day. The next treatment phase was to desensitize patient's nervous system so that she would not get migraines so easily. I checked her sublingual vein, which I found to be enlarged and looked purple. She also had had varicose veins removed surgically a few years earlier. The above vein problems indicated blood stasis due to pregnancy and hormone imbalance. In this case, relying on acupuncture only once a week is not sufficient to get rid of migraines. In addition, I recommended that patient also take herbs. She stopped drinking wine except for minimal consumption at social events. Patient started with a herbal formula twice a day. Miraculously, she did not have any migraines for two months with just once-a-month acupuncture treatments. Patient then changed to once-a-day herbal intake. She also started eating every four hours, having fruit snacks in between the meals, and very little chocolate. Patient did not have migraines for 4 months.

With the onset of the winter holidays, patient came in with a severe migraine, and wanted to continue her Chinese herbs. I asked patient if she would like to try acupuncture with electrical current on her pain areas and certain gallbladder points, and she agreed to the recommendation. I connected GB8 and GV20 with intermittent frequency for 30 min. Patient reported to me subsequently that this was the first time that the migraine stopped right before it became worse, without any medications.

In this case, low blood sugar, alcohol, dehydration, neck muscle tightness and indigestion are factors which can induce or make the migraine worse. Improving her digestion, circulation and balancing her hormones after menopause helped her get rid of her migraines.

A migraine is a type of headache often characterized by a throbbing, stabbing pain occurring on either one or both sides of the head. Migraines can become seriously debilitating for whom ever has them and can also be a chronic, recurring condition. Migraines can occur when abnormal brain cell activities trigger the release of certain chemicals, causing changes of blood flow in the brain and surrounding tissues. CT's or MRI's do not show any organic changes in the brain.

The most prominent symptom of a migraine is a pulsating, throbbing pain that occurs on one side or both sides of the head (though it can be worse on one side). The pain usually lasts between 4 to 72 hours and can become worse with activities that require exertion, such as climbing stairs. Similarly, the pain can be reduced by relaxing and lying down.

Other symptoms that can accompany the pain include:

1.   Nausea and vomiting
2.   Chills
3.   Neck pain
4.   Increased urination
5.   Numbness and tingling

6. Abnormal sweating

7. Sleepiness and dulled thinking

8. Vision changes that include seeing wavy lines or dots and flashing lights, blurry vision, and eye pain.

Causes of migraines:

1. A changed sleep-wake cycle can cause an imbalance of chemicals in the brain. If cortisol, melatonin and other chemicals peak and drop at the wrong times, brain activity will change.

2. Artificial light, such as computer and TV light, can reduce melatonin secretion, which is associated with the hyper-excitability of brain cells and increases of certain chemicals linked with pain sensation. Many teenagers develop migraines after prolonged screen time.

3. Missing meals can cause a decrease in blood sugar, triggering adrenaline release and changing the activity of brain cells.

4. Strong coffee or tea can over-stimulate the sympathetic nervous system and lead to an imbalance between excitatory and inhibitory chemicals in the brain.

5. Taking medication for headaches daily can profoundly change the balance of the chemicals in the body.

6. Hormone changes during puberty, menopause and menstruation can also influence brain blood flow. Women tend to develop migraines during menopause.

7. Birth control pills not only dramatically change your chemical balance and brain activities but can also cause swelling in blood vessels, leading to migraines.

8. Certain smells or perfumes can change blood vessel tone (constriction).

9. Certain foods: any processed, fermented, pickled, or marinated foods, baked goods, chocolate, dairy products, foods containing monosodium glutamate (MSG), foods containing tyramine (including red wine, aged cheese, smoked fish, chicken livers, figs, and certain beans.), meats containing nitrates (bacon, hot dogs, salami, cured meats), nuts, onions and peanut butter.

10. Stress can cause increases of cortisol, adrenaline and prolactin, causing migraines.

11. Lyme disease can cause nerve damage.

12. Dehydration induces histamine release, which generally causes inflammation and dilation of the blood vessels, thus causing migraines.

13. Some medications, such as beta-blockers, can cause swelling in blood vessels.

14. Excessive noise can over-stimulate the sympathetic nervous system, making you prone to developing migraines.

15. Pregnant women may have migraine attacks during the last two trimesters due to high levels of progesterone and a certain type of estrogen (estriol) changing the activities of the blood vessels.

16.   Nicotine withdrawal can cause headaches.

17.   Weather changes may cause swelling of the blood vessels due to changes of humidity and air pressure.

What can you do to prevent migraines?

1.   Go to sleep and wake up at regular, consistent times in order to maintain normal brain cell activity. Healthy individuals typically maintain a proper circadian cycle.

2.   Avoid too much caffeine. If you currently have a migraine, you should gradually cut down the amount of caffeine that you take in. Technically, caffeine can constrict the blood vessels and help relieve headaches if you do not drink coffee regularly. Too much caffeine is always linked with frequent headaches, because caffeine can also over stimulate your sympathetic nervous system, causing overreactions to environmental changes. Moderation is the key.

3.   If you want to quit smoking, do it gradually, because a sudden drop in nicotine can lead to hyper excitability of brain cells. Consider drinking some green tea when you want to light a cigarette, because theanine in green tea can help us relax but still stay alert.

4.   Cut down on alcohol consumption if you have frequent migraines, it interferes with the effectiveness of migraine medication.

5.	Stay away from foods you may be allergic to, such as nuts or onions. Abnormal levels of histamine due to allergies can change our brain cell activities causing migraine.

6.	Avoid intense exercise, which can trigger adrenaline release and cause migraines.

7.	Avoid artificial sweeteners, as they can have similar structures as certain brain chemicals such as aspartate or glutamate and thus can potentially change brain cell activities.

8.	Try to maintain proper blood sugar levels by eating at consistent times. Cut down on foods, such as sweets, that can cause your blood sugar levels to rise and drop rapidly.

9.	Apply a cool towel to your head during a migraine, which can help to reduce blood vessel swelling.

10.	Drink half your weight in fluid ounces of water at least three times a week. When you are dehydrated, your blood vessels tend to constrict to maintain your blood pressure. Furthermore, dehydration can induce histamine release.

Research about acupuncture and migraine:

As reported in 2009, in Military Medicine publication, researcher applied a set of standardized acupuncture points, over a predetermined time interval, on 26 subjects suffering from chronic daily headaches, the majority being migraines. Researchers observed a reduction in the frequency and intensity of headaches, after treatment, as reflected below:

Headache calendars and validated measurements were compared 12 weeks before and 12 weeks after the acupuncture intervention. The outcome reflected continued improvements lasting beyond 12 weeks after the last acupuncture treatment. In another study published in Acupoints' Dictionary of the People's Republic of China, 275 migraine patients admitted to 3 hospitals were randomly divided into a treatment group treated by EA at Qiuxu (GB 40), and a control group treated by EA at Tian shu (ST 25). The indexes of the migraine symptoms and the 5-HT (serotonin) levels were observed in both groups before and after treatment. There was a significant difference in pain score between the two groups ($P < 0.01$). The pain score was much lower in the treatment group than in the control group. Right after treatment and 3 months after the acupuncture treatment, the effective rates were 68.0% and 68.0% in the treated group (ES on GB40) and 24.0% and 32.0% in the control group, and the differences between the two groups were statistically significant. The evidence proves that acupuncture preventive treatments can effectively improve the quality of life of patients with migraine and reduce the frequency of migraine attacks.

Li Y published results in *Headache* in 2009 reflecting how acupuncture can relieve the acute attacks of migraines. A total of 218 patients with migraine were recruited for the study; 180 met the inclusion criteria; 175 completed the callback process and were randomized into 3 groups. One group received true acupuncture, whereas subjects in the other 2 groups were treated with sham acupuncture. Each patient received 1 session of treatment and was observed over a period of 24 hours. The primary outcome measure was the differences in visual analog scale (VAS) scores for the pain level before treatment, and in intervals of 0.5, 1, 2, and 4 hours after treatment. VAS is used to measure the pain level from no pain to worse pain by making a handwritten mark on a 10-cm line. There was a significant difference in the change from baseline in VAS scores in the second hour after treatment among the 3 groups (P = .006), with only patients treated with real acupuncture showing a significant mean decrease in VAS score at this time, Significant differences were observed in pain relief, relapse, or aggravation within 24 hours after treatment as well as in the general evaluations among the 3 groups. Many patients in the acupuncture group experienced complete pain relief (40.7%) and did not experience recurrence or intensification of pain (79.6%). Using

Positron emission computerized tomography, Li XZ observed the changes of glucose metabolism in the brains of patients suffering with migraine before and after acupuncture. Six cases of chronic migraine were treated with acupuncture at Fengchi (GB 20), Waiguan (TE 5), Yang-lingquan (GB 34) on the Shaoyang Channel. After acupuncture, the activities of brain regions associated with pain sensation, such as the brain stem and insula, were reduced, including both temporal lobes. When the neurons are not hypersensitive, the pain threshold can be elevated and the pain sensation can be lowered. Acupuncture achieves beneficial therapeutic effects possibly through coordination and redistribution of energy metabolism in the brain.

Chapter

Fourteen

Sleep Apnea

S leep apnea is the cessation of breathing that occurs during sleep from obstruction of the airway or from the inability of the brain to initiate respiration. The cause of the complete or partial obstruction of the airway is unclear, but it is said that in most people, the site of the obstruction is the soft palate and that people with sleep apnea relax their muscles so much during sleep that their airways collapse. Common among adults, this condition affects as many as 12 million people. If sleep apnea goes untreated, it may lead to serious health consequences such as cardiovascular diseases, weight gain, high blood pressure, impotence, memory loss, and headaches due to the prolonged lack of oxygen.

Clinical Case Study for Sleep Apnea

FM, a Vietnam War veteran, came to see me with a couple of complaints: pain in his right hip, his neck, and lower back, sleep apnea, and the claustrophobia he developed during the War. Although he used to eat a lot of sweet, salty, and greasy foods, he changed his diet after reading a book about the evils of sugar. Despite his upbringing in a Middle Eastern family, he also stopped drinking coffee a long time ago. By his strong will, he developed a very healthy lifestyle, maintaining good energy and strong motivation.

As he does much physical labor working construction, his hip and neck probably developed osteoarthritis due to daily wear and tear. Because he had very healthy nerves and blood vessels due to his healthy diet, his hip condition improved quickly after I treated him with acupuncture four times.

We then started focusing more on his sleep apnea. I examined his throat and found neither inflammation nor phlegm. Although he could sleep on his side without problems, if he accidentally rolled over onto his back, he would sometimes stop breathing, suddenly wake up, and jump out of bed, panting with a rapidly beating heart. This overreaction indicates that his sympathetic nervous system is very sensitive, even to trivial stimulants.

Because FM works very hard during the day and never takes a nap, at night, he sleeps very deeply, and his airway constricts during this deep sleep. When he rolls over on his back, his airway narrows even more due to the increased function of his parasympathetic nerves and the collapse of his soft palate. If his blood oxygen concentration drops below a certain threshold, his sympathetic system reacts so strongly that he jumps out of his bed, feeling like he is about to suffocate.

In this case, phlegm is not an issue; we just needed to desensitize the sympathetic nervous system. I told him to practice lying on his back before he gets up from bed and when he benches weights. We also tried some acupuncture points on his back for the same purpose. After two weeks, he discovered that when he rolls over onto his back, he no longer has to jump out of bed instantly. The imbalance of FM's nervous system is connected with insufficient levels of relaxing neurotransmitters, such as serotonin and GABA. Even though he eats very healthily, he works so hard during the day that he depletes his relaxing neurotransmitters, causing increased sympathetic activity even at night. When his oxygen level drops, instead of breathing harder, he reacts in the "fight or flight" fashion. One of the best ways to correct this problem is to take a nap and meditate for 20 minutes every day so that he can strengthen the relaxing part of his nervous system in order to produce more balanced hormones levels and prevent sleep apnea.

Have you ever noticed that when some people lie down, their faces become red and flushed and their stomachs and intestines make regular noises? These reactions indicate that the parasympathetic nervous system becomes stronger when people are relaxing or sleeping. As we get older, the parasympathetic nervous system weakens and our muscles lose their tone so we tend to develop sleep apnea.

232

Why do we snore?

When our airway is blocked, our blood oxygen level quickly drops, which stimulates our nervous system to breathe harder to open up the airway, creating noise. If our blood oxygen level drops too low, damage to our nerve cells and heart function will occur. Brain death may even occur if we do not get sufficient oxygen for more than 10 minutes.

Why is sleep apnea so common?

1. Obesity: An excess of fat surrounding the neck may cause obstructions to happen more readily and more frequently.

2. Inflammation of the throat: If a person has acute or chronic inflammation of the throat, the narrowing of the airway that causes him to clear his throat to eliminate trapped phlegm in the daytime very likely triggers sleep apnea at night. During sleep, as the parasympathetic nervous system reenergizes, the trachea narrows even further, triggering snoring and sleep apnea. Lying face up especially enhances the parasympathetic nervous system because there are many acupuncture points on the back that strengthen its function. Moreover, throat muscles relax the most when lying face up, further blocking the airway and lowering the concentration of blood oxygen. Snoring ensues to widen the airway. If the blood oxygen concentration continues to drop below acceptable levels, the body triggers an adrenaline release, causing

sudden reactions such as jumping out of bed to resume breathing and increasing heart rate dramatically in the "fight or flight" response.

3. Extreme fatigue: If you are exhausted, you may sleep very deeply. Your parasympathetic nervous system becomes much stronger than your sympathetic nervous system, so your trachea constricts more than usual, narrowing your airway.

4. Altered hormone levels: Pregnant women tend to snore, underscoring the relationship between phlegm and sleep apnea. When women get pregnant, their estrogen and progesterone levels increase sharply, so they tend to retain fluids in different areas of the body. In the lower leg, their ankles may become swollen; in the throat, they may develop a lot of phlegm. In addition, high progesterone relaxes smooth muscles such as the uterus, stomach, bladder, and soft palate. All these factors can contribute to the narrowing of the airway when women sleep on their backs.

5. Loss of muscle tone: Aging lowers growth and other hormone levels, which leads to muscle drooping.

6. Imbalanced nervous system: When people take drugs to treat certain neurological diseases such as epilepsy, their parasympathetic nervous system, artificially enhanced by the medication, can cause sleep apnea.

How can we treat sleep apnea?

Positional Therapy: Try to sleep on your side. You can put a tennis ball in a tube sock and pin the sock to the back of your pajamas to prevent yourself from sleeping face-up. You can also elevate your upper back to open up your airway more. However, these methods may cause neck muscle tightness or even spasms, so you need to stretch your muscles before going to sleep and after getting up in the morning.

Avoid alcohol and nervous system suppressants such as painkillers, sedatives and muscle relaxants: These can reduce the breathing drive in your brain and cause the airway to collapse by upsetting the balance of the nervous system.

Oral appliances: Oral appliances prevent the tongue from falling back into the airway or push the lower jaw forward to open the airway more. However, not everybody can tolerate these devices and a few people may even have worse sleep apnea after using them.

Surgery: Surgery can remove the excess tissues around the airway or harden the soft palate by inserting three polyester rods. The buildup of scar tissues, however, may lead to other problems in the future.

Weight loss: Weight loss can reduce the fat around the airway so that, when sleeping, the airway will not collapse completely.

Exercise: Toning your neck muscles by doing exercises such as sit-ups every day can help.

Continuous Positive Airway Pressure Mask: This device can be used as a splint to keep the airway open by blowing room air through the airway at a pressure high enough to keep the throat open. The pressure can be adjusted according to each individual but some people can never get used to sleeping with this mask.

If you practice a healthy lifestyle and have no inflammation or phlegm accumulating in your throat, the above methods may help you achieve better sleep. If inflammation and phlegm continue to sensitize your throat, however, you may be unable to tolerate the treatments above, which is why some people get better results than others.

How can we prevent throat inflammation and reduce phlegm?

1. Reduce your salt intake: If you eat very salty foods, you should drink enough water to discharge the extra sodium and thereby avoid water retention and phlegm.

2. Do not eat too many sweets: According to Chinese medicine, sweets can impede digestion and produce phlegm in different parts of the body. I had a very interesting experience last fall when I allowed myself to have a piece of dark chocolate before jogging with my daughter, thinking that I would burn off the calories by exercising. I was in a

hurry, so I did not drink any water. Two hours after finishing my jog in the windy and cold weather, I completely lost my voice and had to find someone to substitute for me at the acupuncture school the next day. It took me several days to regain my voice by taking Chinese herbs. In my case, chocolate dehydrated my throat, stimulating the release of histamine, which led to swelling and inflammation. As a child, I used to have throat infections repeatedly and lost my voice at least twice a year. In the winter, I had to wear a mask when jogging to avoid laryngitis. Whenever I did get laryngitis, I would have to take antibiotics for a week and then wait another two weeks to recover. These repeated infections sensitized my throat, causing chronic inflammation so that in my adult life, whenever I have any sweets, salty foods, or alcohol, I would immediately develop phlegm in my throat.

3. Avoid spicy food: Spicy food generally produces heat and dries up body fluids, causing inflammation in the throat. In this society, we tend to overeat food that stimulates our taste buds, because we have so much food and so much freedom to eat whenever and whatever we want. When I treat esophagus and stomach cancer patients, I always ask them if they used to eat a lot of spicy food, and the answer is always yes. If you follow people who overeat spicy food, you will find that they eventually develop inflammation somewhere in their bodies.

4. Do not take anti-histamines for more than a month: Anti-histamines stop membrane secretion, causing you to have an extremely dry throat.

Long-term use may lead to the loss of your voice or permanent damage to your vocal cords. An opera singer I treated took β-blockers to lower her blood pressure and ended up with a lot of phlegm in her throat. She began using anti-histamines regularly and, after a couple of years, she could not sing any more.

5. Avoid consuming too many dairy products: Dairy products can also trigger the body to produce a lot of phlegm.

Some people diagnosed with sleep apnea have neither chronic inflammation nor phlegm in their throats. This kind of sleep apnea may be associated with an imbalance of the autonomic nervous system. S.V. Somers et al. of the University Of Iowa College Of Medicine recorded blood pressure, heart rate, sympathetic nerve activity, and brain activity during wakefulness and sleep in 10 patients with obstructive sleep apnea. The above measurements were also obtained from four patients after treatments with an oxygen mask. In addition, sympathetic activity was measured during wakefulness in 10 control subjects and 5 obese subjects without histories of sleep apnea.

Patients with sleep apnea had high levels of sympathetic nerve activity even when asleep. Their blood pressure and sympathetic activity, which increased especially during stage II and REM sleep, did not fall during any stage of sleep. Wearing a continuous positive airway pressure (CPAP) oxygen mask at night, however, decreased their sympathetic activity and blood pressure. The researchers concluded that patients with obstructive sleep apnea have abnormally high sympathetic activity when awake and further increases in blood pressure and sympathetic activity during certain stages of sleep. Thus, when their airway is blocked and their blood oxygen level drops, they may suddenly jump out of bed in a "fight or flight" response.

Why should we prevent sleep apnea?

Clinical Studies published in Journal of The American College of Cardiology in 1999, suggest that people who have sleep apnea have an increased risk for ischemic heart disease. Habitual snoring is also associated with increased risk of sudden death during sleep. In patients with severe obstructive sleep apnea, there is reasonable evidence to indicate a high mortality rate in the absence of treatments. Death is predominantly due to cardiovascular problems and tends to occur during sleep because the lowered oxygen level can cause permanent damage to brain and heart tissue.

F. Jurysta of the Free University of Brussels, Belgium, studied the autonomic cardiac control during different stages of sleep in people with sleep apnea. He agrees that sleep apnea is related to cardiovascular complications and that those with sleep apnea show higher sympathetic activity than normal subjects during sleep. In healthy people, non-rapid eye movement (NREM) sleep is associated with decreased heart rate and blood pressure, whereas rapid eye movement (REM) sleep is linked to cardiac sympathetic activity, in which blood pressure and heart rate rise. Those with sleep apnea demonstrate a loss of fluctuations in cardiac autonomic activity, so their heart rate and blood pressure do not go down even when they enter deep sleep. Therefore, their heart never has the chance to rest and repair itself.

Acupuncture and sleep apnea:

As reported in Sleep Medicine 2007, researchers in Brazil investigated the efficacy of acupuncture in the treatment of moderate obstructive sleep apnea syndrome through a randomized, placebo-controlled, single-blinded study, with blinded evaluation. 36 patients presenting with sleep apnea/hypopnea were randomly assigned to three groups: 12 acupuncture, 12 sham (needle insertion in non-acupoints), and 12 control (no treatment). Patients received acupuncture or sham acupuncture once a week for 10 weeks. Upon completion of the study, the number of occurrences of breathing cessation decreased significantly in the acupuncture group but not in the sham group. On the other hand, the control group displayed significant deterioration in some polysomnographic parameters and a significant increase in the number of breathing changes. Acupuncture treatment significantly improved (before vs. after treatment) the patients' functional quality of life and excessive daytime sleepiness.

In the Journal of Traditional Chinese Medicine 2009, Dr. XH Wang et al. used auricular plaster therapy in which the needles or ear pressing ball to reduce respiratory and sleep disturbances. Auricular plaster therapy showed good therapeutic affects for sleep apnea with low cost and very few side effects. Another group of Chinese researchers found that acupuncture can increase blood oxygen saturation in patients with sleep apnea.

The most popular treatment for sleep apnea is the continuous positive airway pressure (CPAP) oxygen mask. One group of researchers compared the effects of acupuncture and nasal continuous positive airway pressure (nCPAP) on obstructive sleep apnea-hypopnea syndrome (OSAHS). 66 sleep apnea patients were randomly divided into an acupuncture group treated at the acupoints Lianquan (CV 23) and Tianrong (SI 17) and an nCPAP group. Respiration rate, blood oxygen level, and sleep were monitored before, during, and after treatment. Compared with before treatment, no significant differences in maximum apnea duration, sleep time spent with O_2 saturation below 90%, and the micro arousal index were found in the acupuncture group during treatment, but these indices improved significantly at the end of treatment. Although the therapeutic effect of nCPAP was better than that of acupuncture during the treatment period, no significant differences in therapeutic effects were found at the end of the treatment period and the benefits of acupuncture outlasted that of nCPAP. On one hand, although oxygen therapy can give instant relief, the effects gradually disappear. On the other, acupuncture provides longer lasting results but patients should expect to complete at least 12 to 24 treatments before obtaining good results.

Acupuncture points for sleep apnea:

Fengfu (GV 16): On the back of the neck, 1.0 cun directly above the midpoint of the posterior hairline.

Yamen (GV 15): On the back of the neck, 0.5 cun directly above the midpoint of the posterior hairline.

Fengchi (GB20): In the depression posterior and inferior to the mastoid process.

CV23: In the depression above the upper border of the hyoid bone.

SI17: In the posterior border of m. sternocleidomastoideus, at the same level with the Adam's apple.

LI18: At the same level of the Adam's apple between the sternal head and clavicular head of m. sternocleidomastoideus.

Chinese Herbal Remedies for sleep apnea:

1. Phlegm obstructs the airway:

Symptoms: Constantly clearing the throat, tendency to eat salty foods and a lot of dairy products or meat. Snoring reduced if patient drinks more water, fatigue after 8 hour sleep, heavy sensation. Tongue: Swollen with a watery or white greasy coating. Pulse: Soggy or slippery.

Herbal formula: Jiang Ban Xia 9g, Chen Pi 6g, Dan Nan Xing 9g, Gua Lou 15g, Fu Ling 20g, Zhi Gan Cao 6g, Yi Yi Ren 20g, Jie Geng 6g.

2. Heat blocked in upper burner:

Symptoms: Tendency to over think, cannot sit down and relax, always multi-tasking, cold hands and feet, sensitivity to environmental changes, and tendency to develop anxiety, panic attacks, and insomnia. Tongue: Red tip with thin yellow or white coating. Pulse: Thin and wiry.

Herbal formula: Dan Zhu Ye 12g, Lian Zi Xin 15g, Zhi Zi 6g, Huang Qin 6g, Dan Dou Chi 6g, Sheng Di 9g. Sheng Long Gu 15g, Sheng Mu Li 15g, Xiang Fu 12g.

Chapter 15

Cystitis

ystitis is the inflammation of the urinary bladder and the ureters. The Symptoms are frequent and urgent urination, lower abdominal pressure and pain, and sometimes pain in the vagina and urethra, which can range from a mild burning or discomfort to severe pain.

Mechanism of Cystitis: The protective mucous membrane inside the bladder is damaged, so urine can irritate and inflame the bladder lining. If the concentration or the acidity of urine is too high, the mucous membrane cannot protect the bladder any more.

Cystitis Case Study:

This case study reminded me of some important truths. As we age, our bodies react differently to our medications, diet and lifestyle. What used to be OK for a 21 year old, can create medical problems for someone who is a bit older. Secondly, everyone's body is different, so the remedy for a disease such as cystitis might be unique for each person based on their social and medical history and DNA. So there might not be a single pill to take that fixes your unique experience. And thirdly, the road to being 100% healthy might not be straight. I might cure a remote problem: e.g. hormone balance or body acidity, etc that leads to the cure of the original symptoms identified. We treat the person, not so much the disease. This person is made of interdependent systems that want to be normal again. It may not be one root cause, but a tweaking of a bodily process. I hope you will see what I mean as you read the story of LZ.

LZ is a nurse who used to drink a lot of coffee to maintain her alertness in order to take good care of her patients. Like many other American women, she started taking birth control pills when she was just a teenager to control her heavy period and acne. The pill reduced her heavy blood flow during her period and made her skin very smooth. Seven years ago, however, after she passed 40, she was diagnosed with intestinal cystitis exhibiting frequent and urgent urination and abdominal pressure, burning sensations, and chronic vulvar pain when she urinated. Furthermore, her periods became heavier and her menstrual cramps returned despite continuing to take the birth control pill.

She went to see different medical specialists and was told to stop eating acidic food. First, she gave up coffee, then, all fruits except bananas, blueberries, and pears. Her frequent urination woke her up every hour at night, interrupting her sleep and making her exhausted during the day. She started drinking 10 cups of peppermint tea a day, hoping that she would not have a sudden drop in energy in the afternoon while working at the hospital. Initially, her symptoms only worsened two weeks before her period, although three days after her period, she could almost feel normal.

Despite taking anti-inflammatory medications for a year, when she first visited me, she still needed to urinate every hour with excruciating pain. Her pain became so bad right before the period and immediately after that she had to wear a lidocaine patch at work. Interestingly, the vulva pain becomes less when she lay down.

In my opinion, she developed inflammation in her bladder due to a hormone imbalances caused by aging and long-term usage of the birth control pill. She did not drink enough water so the concentrated minerals from her tea stimulated her bladder lining, causing it to become inflamed and very sensitive. Her deficiency of vitamins and potassium resulting from prolonged intake of the pill aggravated the typical imbalance of estrogen and progesterone around menopause, leading to a progressive worsening of her symptoms. Because the birth control pill had manipulated her hormones for 25 years, her unnatural hormone levels also threw her immune function off balance and sensitized her nerves. These imbalances explain why her symptoms increased two weeks before her period when her estrogen went up too high and right after her period when her progesterone suddenly dropped too low. With her cycle reset every 28 days, she has very few days of comfort.

My first step was to convince her to replace her tea with at least 8 cups of water per day. I told her that this increased water intake would not make her frequent urination at night worse since she already got up every one or two hours to urinate anyway. On the other hand, more water would dilute any stimulating chemicals in her urine and help discharge toxic materials from her body, especially the metabolites of estrogen. To balance her estrogen and progesterone, she needed to stop taking the birth control pill. Her period became heavier despite the pill after she gave birth to her two children, indicating that her estrogen level was too high relative to progesterone. Furthermore, she had suffered from severe breast tenderness for the past two years, another sign of hormone imbalance.

She followed my advice and she did not drink any tea for a week. On the first day, she still experienced pain upon urination and felt exhausted. Then, on the second day, she slept for 4 hours without getting up and even felt completely normal when she awoke. Despite stopping the birth control pill, she got her period on time and felt much better on the first day of menstruation whereas in the past she suffered from severe pain for 3 to 4 days. When she lay down, she had no pain at all and she had more energy than before.

We continued acupuncture treatments and gradually she could lie down with needles in her back and lower abdomen for 30 minutes. She could also empty her bladder more than before, which allowed her to hold urine longer. However, her vulva pain still came and went, so we decided to stop her anti-inflammatory medications, using herbs instead to balance her hormones and immune function. After ten days, just before getting her period, she experienced almost no pain. If she stood and worked long hours, her vulva pain would return, but this problem could be quickly resolved by sitting down or drinking more water. Since her bladder lining was still fragile and the nerves controlling the bladder and pelvic muscle were sensitive, she needed to continue taking herbs for 3 to 6 months to get rid of the inflammation and hormone imbalance. At this point, the occasional pain did not interrupt her work and her sleep had become deeper. Because at her age, ovarian function is changing every day and because she worked in a highly stressful environment, she continues with the herbs to reduce her stress and to restore her balance.

In LZ's case, initially the anti-inflammatory medications helped mitigate her inflammation and she felt better. When she passed 40 years old, however, her adrenal and ovarian functions declined, so although her medications stayed the same, her body could not compensate any more. Had she not stopped the birth control pill, her imbalanced immune function could have led to other autoimmune diseases.

248

Although the peppermint tea she drank is generally good for the body, because of her inflamed bladder lining, it became harmful. Once her body got rid itself of the inflammation, she was able to resume drinking 1 to 2 cups of tea. Moderation is the key for the happier and healthier life.

What can cause inflammation of the bladder?

1.   Hormone imbalance before, during, and after menopause: When estrogen is not balanced with progesterone, mast cells in bladder tissue are easily activated to release many kinds of chemicals that cause inflammation in those tissues, as discovered by researchers from Tufts Medical School in 1998. This is one of the reasons why women between 35 and 55 tend to develop cystitis if they do not eat a balanced diet.

2.   Imbalanced nervous system: When you get nervous, you tend to use the bathroom more than you should. In addition, the nervous system regulates immune cell activities and the magnitude of the immune response. If immune function is hyperactive from the overstimulation of the sympathetic nervous system, then inflammation in the bladder will become chronic. That is why relaxation and meditation help balance your immune function.

3.   Chronic stress: Stress depletes our anti-inflammatory hormones such as cortisol. When I was supervising the Chinese Herbal

Clinic at the New England School of Medicine, I met a young lady who developed interstitial cystitis presenting constant lower abdominal pressure, an urgency to urinate, and a burning sensation in the urethra that dramatically interfered with her life. Even though she visited many hospitals and physicians and underwent extensive tests, no one could determine what caused these problems. She tried many kinds of medications, but nothing worked. I discussed with her about factors that might trigger this disease under certain conditions. She said that at the time, she had tremendous stress and one day drank 10 cups of coffee to try to work more hours. Shortly afterwards, she developed this disease. In this case, stress initially stimulated her adrenal gland to produce more endogenous cortisol. Then, too much caffeine stimulated her sympathetic nervous system to produce more adrenaline. Finally, the adrenal gland, depleted by the great amount of caffeine she took in short period of time, could no longer protect her from inflammation. Although our bodies have a tremendous ability to compensate, if abused for too long, it will eventually fail us.

4.   Feminine hygiene sprays and spermicidal jellies: These products can cause inflammation when your immune system is already out of balance, which is why not every woman will develop cystitis from using the same product for the same period of the time. If

you currently have bladder inflammation, try to avoid these products until your symptoms are gone.

5.   Carbonated beverages: Carbonated beverages create an acidic environment in the body, which facilitates inflammation. If the inflammation occurs in the bladder, then you may develop cystitis.

6.   Caffeine: Caffeine aggravates the symptoms of cystitis according to a 2005 article from the Journal of the British Menopause Society. Caffeine not only creates an acidic environment in the body, but also causes an imbalance of the immune and nervous systems.

7.   Citrus products: Most articles blame citrus products for causing inflammation of the bladder, but I think that the vitamin C in citrus actually helps our body build stronger connective tissues. I used to have canker sores regularly a week before my period started and they would last for two weeks, causing me severe pain. Since I began eating one orange or tangerine a day, I have not had this problem for a long time. Moreover, oranges help our digestion, so that our body can absorb other nutrients more efficiently. If people eat citrus while drinking soda or coffee, however, their bodies cannot buffer the acidity so inflammation then occurs. Finally, I do not think that orange juice provides the same benefits as actual oranges.

8. Alcohol: Alcohol inflames your digestive membranes, causing vitamin and mineral deficiency. Your body, including the bladder, cannot repair itself without sufficient vitamins and minerals even if you take multi-vitamins every day. Alcohol can also cause urine retention, which leads to damage of the bladder lining.

9. Spicy food: Spicy food can cause acute urine retention and inflammation because it irritates the bladder lining especially if you eat too much of it, too frequently, and without drinking enough water.

10. Artificial sweetener: The Mayo Clinic recommends that women who have cystitis avoid artificial sweeteners. Artificial sweeteners can inflame the small nerves of the bladder, making your bladder hypersensitive.

11. Radiation: Radiation therapy can cause inflammation of the bladder and its controlling nerves.

12. Catheters: Long-term use of a catheter can cause the inflammation and even infection of bladder and urethra linings.

13. Autoimmune reaction: If a person has an autoimmune disease, such as lupus, MS, or colitis, his/her immune system produces different kinds of antibodies that attack the tissues and lead to chronic inflammation.

14. Allergies: When you have allergies, your mast cells produce more of the chemicals associated with chronic inflammation, including

histamine. In this case, using herbs to resolve your allergies as soon as possible will help relieve your cystitis.

15. Bacteria: Bacterial infection can cause chronic inflammation of the bladder.

16. Certain drugs: Ryanodine, heparin, 2-aminoethoxydiphenyl, atropin, belladonna, efedrin, aminasin, tizercin, phenobarbital, imisin, promedol, and lazix can cause urine retention. Because the urine becomes more concentrated, the bladder is more prone to inflammation.

17. Avoid eating too much canned meat, aged cheese, and fish.

18. Onions, fava beans, and spinach can irritate the bladder lining.

19. Avoid most nuts including pine nuts and almonds when you have cystitis.

What should we do to make our bladders healthy?

1. Quite smoking.

2. Cut down or stop drinking alcohol during flare ups of cystitis. Once the symptoms are gone, you may try drinking moderately once or twice week.

3. Wear loose cotton clothes. Synthetic materials usually cause irritation and cannot absorb sweat as easily. The resulting damp environment helps bacteria and fungi grow.

4. Bladder training: You should go to the bathroom at regular intervals instead of waiting until you feel really uncomfortable. If

you hold your urine too long, it becomes more concentrated and the harmful materials in it may be more likely to irritate your bladder lining.

5. Reduce your stress level with acupuncture, yoga, tai chi, and meditation: Less stress means that you will have more anti-inflammatory hormones to protect your bladder lining.

6. The Kegel Exercise for bladder control: Tighten your pelvic muscles by stopping urine flow. Count to 10 and then, relax those muscles by restarting urine flow. Practice this exercise 3 times a day.

7. Eat wheat grass, green barley, alfalfa, kelp, and seaweed. These foods will create an alkaline condition in your body, thus reducing bladder inflammation.

8. Eat cantaloupe, melons, and pears, which can help clear internal heat and reduce inflammation according to Chinese medical theory.

9. Avoid onions, tofu, soybeans, lima beans, fava beans, yogurt, sour cream, nuts (except almonds and pine nuts) and foods containing nitrates and preservatives when you have interstitial cystitis because they can modify your immune function and estrogen activity. You may resume eating small amounts of these foods after your cystitis heals.

10. Drink enough water to flush out your urethra and bladder. Water also helps lower your histamine level, thus reducing

inflammation. Do not be afraid of frequent urination. The less water you drink the more irritation your bladder feels because the toxins in your urine are more concentrated. If you make a chart of how many times you urinate each day compared to your water intake, you may find that your urination frequency is almost the same regardless of how much water you drink. However, avoid drinking water after 7 PM to prevent urination from disrupting your sleep.

11.   Food supplements: Calcium glycerophosphate, L-arginine, mucopolysaccharides, and bioflavinoids can help repair damaged tissues in the bladder. Co-enzyme Q (200 mg) and vitamin E (400 IU) have strong antioxidant effects, thus helping reduce tissue damage.

Foods for treating and preventing interstitial cystitis:

Many very safe Chinese herbs, which can help your body balance the immune and nervous systems to reduce chronic inflammation, are also edible as food.

1.   Improve lung and kidney function, optimize the digestive function, and reduce the frequency of urination. Steam wild yam and eat about 30 g per day.

2.   Dandelions greens: Helps clear internal heat to reduce inflammation and also cleanse the liver. Stir fry them with olive oil.

3.   Bitter melon: Helps clear internal heat. Stir-fry it with olive oil.

4.   Honeysuckleflowers: Has anti-inflammatory effects. Soak the flowers in hot water for 5 to 10 minutes and drink as tea.

5.   Parsley: Helps neutralize your body fluids so that they are neither too acidic nor basic. Put parsley into your soup.

Why acupuncture helps relieve the symptoms of cystitis:

1.   Acupuncture can relax your bladder and pelvic floor muscles so that they do not contract constantly when the bladder is not yet full.

2.   Acupuncture can desensitize the nerves controlling the bladder so that it does not leak small amounts of urine or become so sensitized to the irritating chemicals in the urine.

3.   Acupuncture can relieve pelvic pain by stimulating your body to produce its own painkillers: endorphin, serotonin, and dopamine.

4.   Acupuncture can change your perception of pain so that you focus less on when and how you can get to the bathroom. Furthermore, it reduces the pain signal in the pain processing center of your brain.

Chinese Herbal Remedy:

In Chinese medicine, interstitial cystitis is related to heat in the small intestine and heart channels. The herbs I use to treat this disease have the functions of clearing the heat in both channels and of tonifying the Yin, which diminishes after 35 to 40 years old, in order to rebalance the Yin and Yang.

Herbal formula: Tong Cao 6g, Sheng Di Huang 12g, Dan Zhu Ye 12g, Che Qian Zi 12g, Sheng Gan Cao 6g, Zhi Zi 6g, Chuan Niu Xi 10g, Huang Bai 12g.

Acupuncture points to relieve bladder muscle spasms and inflammation:

1. CV4: 3 cun below the center of the belly button on the front midline. The crossing point of Ren and three foot Yin meridian, the front-mu point of small intestine.

2. Kid11 (Heng Gu): 0.5 cun lateral to the anterior midline, 5 Cun below the belly button, the crossing point of kidney meridian and chong meridian.

3. Liv7 (Zhong Du): 7 cun above the tip of the medial malleolus, on the middle of the medial aspect of the tibia, Xi-cleft point of Liver meridian has homeostatic function, thus help treat acute, painful disease by reducing the inflammation.

Chapter 16

Irregular Heartbeats

I
t might sneak up on you, seemingly out of nowhere. This ailment has surprised my patients who have been athletes, soldiers, and women who have run marathons. They have been vigilant people who have been careful about their diet, always the ones to sacrifice sweets, to lay off the salt, and to have small portions. Why then are they the afflicted? We'll get to that later, but for now you should know that it can happen to you. You can be leading a normal life, washing the dishes, walking to your car in the parking lot, selecting groceries at the market. Then what? All of a sudden you feel faint. You get a bit tired too early. You feel something strange in your chest; sometimes your heart runs a little too fast. Sometimes it's fast and then slower. Longer term, your legs can swell. Your doctor might prescribe a beta blocker or coumadin (blood thinner), or worse yet, you might need a pacemaker. It's a problem that many people experience later in life. For women, menopause might trigger it. However, anyone could have irregular heart beat; anytime in their life. I have successfully

treated many people. I have not employed the tools of Western Medicine. I have not installed pacemakers; I have not prescribed beta blockers. I have helped my patients using Chinese Medicine, acupuncture, acupressure and common sense. I will illustrate how by telling the story of my patient, Genevieve Bly.

Genevieve lived on the West Coast, in the Pacific Northwest to be precise. She moved there during the go, go days when Microsoft was starting up. She lived and worked two blocks from the epicenter of all that hoopla. She was a 6th grade teacher there, and she taught the same grade when she moved to Lexington, Massachusetts, and became my patient. Her lifestyle, typical of Seattleites, centered around the caffeine-infused coffee houses, jazz nightclubs, and fast friends; not so typical of a teacher, but Genevieve was different. When I did my first intake, I saw a fit, slim, rather tall brunette. She appeared quick witted, talked fast but seemed remotely troubled. She looked young for her 48 years. I found out over time that this serene looking teacher had a very sensitive autonomic nervous system. Once, during a dental procedure, the epinephrine used to constrict her local blood vessels caused her heart to beat so fast that she was rushed to the emergency room.

She also developed premature ventricular contractions as her menstrual cycle became more irregular. Subsequently, as her daily stress increased, her symptoms worsened. In the follow-up test of a 24-hour EKG, however, there did not appear to be any heart abnormalities. It was surprising to me how calm she appeared as she described all these life changing events. A person could be fooled, but underneath the surface the currents were moving turbulently.

I treated her using two approaches; the first enhanced her ovary and adrenal gland functions so that she could cope better with the physical stress. Furthermore, with enhanced ovarian function, her progesterone level became normal. Since progesterone is a natural body relaxant, her nervous system also became less sensitive to different kinds of environmental stimulations. The second approach was to enhance her parasympathetic nervous system function by stimulating certain points on her feet and back. After 5 acupuncture treatments, her premature ventricular contractions were greatly diminished; her period also started to become more regular.

We stopped treatments for two months during the summer vacation. When school started again, she returned with worse symptoms, even though her periods remained regular. She continued having premature ventricular contractions, especially in the morning when cortisol level goes up. These worsened symptoms seem to have caught her off guard. She was such a fast-moving person that, deep down, I believe she was amazed that something in her own body was slowing her down.

She told me that she drank one cup of coffee after she got up, then went for her workout, and then had her breakfast. I explained to her that when we first get up, our blood sugar level tends to be low; this is true especially for very thin people. If you drink coffee on an empty stomach, it not only quickly stimulates the sympathetic nervous system but also increases insulin levels, which decreases blood sugar levels further. Low blood sugar induces adrenaline release, which also stimulates the sympathetic nervous system. How our body sets the tone of the sympathetic nervous system in the morning will influence the body's balance for the remainder of the day.

Once an irregular heartbeat starts, it tends to continue until we do something to rebalance the two branches of the autonomic nervous system. I told Genevieve that if she was going to run on an empty stomach, then she must drink water instead of coffee. After exercising, she can have both her breakfast and her coffee. I thought she might be able to handle this small change in her life. On the other hand, if a person has an extremely strong parasympathetic nervous system, she usually sleeps so deeply that, in the morning, she will need a cup of coffee to get things going. How a person responds to caffeine or any other kind of stimulant really depends on his or her genetic makeup, stress level, and autonomic nervous system function.

In my practice, I have had several patients who feel very sleepy after drinking coffee. This may sound crazy, but we are all very different physically and mentally. If you feel good after drinking a cup of coffee in the morning, in most cases it will not harm your body. On the other hand, if you have found that it speeds up your heartbeat, causes insomnia, or creates anxiety, panic attacks, then try to substitute it with green tea or decaffeinated coffee.

Genevieve stopped her morning coffee but still ran before breakfast. She continued to have very frequent irregular heartbeats until I finally convinced her to stop running and to try yoga instead. I could have also suggested stretching, qi gong, or tai chi as well, to relieve her stress and calm her sympathetic nervous system. She continued acupuncture treatments while trying to change her exercise routine. After 4 weeks, her premature ventricular contractions completely disappeared.

I am always happy when a good result like this happens. In this case, Genevieve was cured, or so I thought. However, it was short lived. I didn't see her for some time, about 9 months, but one day I received a call for an appointment with no reason given. I at first thought it was a regular rebalancing. That happens with some of my regular patients: no big problem, just a tune up. However, in this case, Genevieve had bad news. Her palpitations had returned about six weeks after she last saw me, and she went to see her general practitioner. He prescribed a beta blocker. That had worked . . . for a couple of months, but now the irregular heartbeat was worse.

She was teary-eyed as she described what she had been through during this long 9 months. She was starting to gain weight in her legs, had less energy, and, scariest of all, she had gone through episodes of her heart beating too fast for no reason, especially in the morning. She had been talking to her doctor, and he had given her some options: blood thinner, and, if that did not work, a pacemaker. She wanted neither; she wanted alternative options, so she had come to me.

She probably had waited too long to come see me. Her symptoms had gotten worse: leg swelling, fatigue, and those very scary moments of irregular heart beating out of control. I wanted her to listen to her doctor first before I began my treatment. It was important to stop the damaging, frequent attacks. I could help her fix this problem long-term, but for now she needed to continue her beta blocker and find out what made her condition worse.

We began a program of no coffee, no wine, light exercise (walking), acupuncture and herbs. My goal was to calm her nervous system enough that she could stop the beta blocker and still be symptom free. After 3 weeks of 2 sessions per week and a prescription of herbs, she accomplished this goal: no beta blocker, no coffee and no symptoms. We continued sessions for 2 months.

At one of the last sessions during this time, she told me she had tried decaffeinated coffee, and her palpitations had returned the next morning. She immediately stopped her little experiment. She substituted black tea with a little milk and was fine. Furthermore, her craving for sweets decreased by drinking black tea and milk. I didn't see her for about 5 months after that, but when she returned, she had a big smile on her face, and her worry lines had disappeared. For some reason during this time, for reasons she did not understand, she had lost 15 pounds. She looked great!

The Science behind My Treatment Methods for Genevieve

What body systems and hormones can affect the beating of your heart?

1. Sympathetic nerves increase heart rate, whereas parasympathetic nerves cause it to decrease.

2. Adrenaline can increase heart rate.

3. When blood pressure drops, heart rate increases automatically.

4. An imbalance of estrogen and progesterone can affect your heart.

5. An imbalance of different hormones and neurotransmitters. For instance, if our calming chemicals, such as GABA or progesterone, are low, the stimulating hormones such as

estrogen, adrenaline and dopamine become relatively stronger. Your nervous system can then become unstable.

What are the daily-life contributors to an irregular heartbeat condition?

1. Caffeine: especially if you drink coffee with an empty stomach in the morning. In Prevention Magazine, there is an article that recommends drinking coffee around 10 to 11 am, after you've had a little breakfast. In most European countries, workers have a coffee break after two hours of work and a full breakfast. In the Chinese tradition, we usually drink tea after a meal, especially after lunch when you feel slightly tired. If you wake up ready to go, you really do not need coffee to stimulate your nervous system. People who wake up from very deep sleep and feel drowsy for the next two hours may use coffee to stimulate their nervous system so that they can get onto the road without causing an accident. When we first get up, our blood cortisol level is rising and our heartbeat is increasing. If you drink coffee on an empty stomach, the stimulating effect is strong and instant, which can set your sympathetic nervous system at a higher tone for the whole day.

2. Low sugar levels stimulate adrenaline release, which also speeds up your heart rate. When you drink coffee on an empty stomach first thing in the morning, the caffeine quickly induces insulin

release, causing a sharp drop in blood sugar. If you run afterwards, the adrenaline rush can make your heart pound even harder with the increased sympathetic activity.

3. Excessive exercising also can induce adrenaline and cortisol release.

4. Sleep deprivation: when you do not get enough sleep, your cortisol level can go up temporarily, which may increase your heart rate. Furthermore, your nervous system becomes more sensitive to environmental changes. I remember that, when I was in my early thirties, whenever I did not sleep enough, I would have an irregular heartbeat. Although I went through various tests, the doctors could never find anything wrong with my heart. However, if sleep deprivation continues for some time, the heart structure may change. Then you may need blood thinner or a pacemaker.

5. Certain medications, such as high dosages of pain killers, can increase your heart rate. A young lady developed severe pain in her vaginal area after she used an over-the-counter anti-yeast cream for a while. The pain was so severe that she could not do her normal work. She was on a very high dosage of painkiller, and her heart rate went up so much that her physician advised her to see Boston Acupuncturist to lower her pain level and heart rate.

How to manage an irregular heartbeat condition?

Breathing exercises: deep breathing in and out at 6 breaths per minute can reduce irregular heartbeat.

Tai Ji: Dr. Jin, in the Journal of Psychosomatic Research (1989), indicates that practicing Tai ji can lower cortisol and adrenalin levels even though your heart rate is slightly elevated during the practice. Therefore, you increase your heart function without increasing your stress hormone level.

Try to avoid constant adrenaline rushes: such as multi-tasking, skipping meals, or having a high sugar diet.

Improve your nerve function: Vitamin B6 helps metabolize amino acids and fat and preserves your nerve function. When people with anxiety are taking antacid medications, they have more frequent panic attacks, combined with racing heartbeats, because their digestive systems cannot absorb vitamins and minerals properly. Older people tend to develop irregular heartbeats if they do not have a proper diet. You might hear your colleagues complain that their parents get very nervous over small things. This happens because, as you age, your digestive system cannot absorb vitamins as efficiently. You may take many kinds of food supplements to provide more vitamins, but if your stomach does not absorb the vitamins efficiently, your nervous system will not be balanced. Foods that are rich in Vitamin B6 are eggs, meat, liver and kidney products, cheese, nuts, whole grains, fish, and potatoes.

The following recipes can be used to calm your nervous system to make your heart healthier:

1. Lung and Heart Qi deficiency:

If you have palpitation: have a very skinny body, very sensitive to temperature changes, have to wear layers of clothes all the time, wake up around 3 to 4 am and feel hot but not sweating, have constipation and dry skin, you may eat this porridge: Add one gallon of filtered water into your crock pot, plus half a cup of brown rice, 1/3 cup of red bean and black bean, Bai Zi Ren30g (Biota Orienalis seed), Long Yan rou20g (Longan Fruit Flesh), set at low grade level, cook overnight. Eat one bowl of this porridge every day, especially in winter.

2. Kidney and Heart Yin deficiency:

If you have palpitation, low back pain, hot flushes, night sweats, feel tired after you run only one mile, and your period is very scanty, you can consume this soup: chicken soup, add Gou

Qi Zi (lycium seed) 12g, lima bean 30g, black bean 30g, Yi Yi Ren 30g, Chinese Yam 30g.

3. Spleen Qi deficiency:

If you tend to have indigestion, bloating, gas or loose stool, with very low stamina, insomnia, heavy period or very light period, and your skin looks yellowish or pale, add dates - 4 pieces, fresh ginger, Yi Yi Ren30g and Chinese Yam 20g in your soup or porridge.

If you have palpitation, with dry throat and coughing, and very dry skin, you can also stir fry Bai He (Lily bulb) with olive oil. You can soak Mai Dong (Ophiopogon) in hot water and seep the water for a whole day.

4. Spleen Qi deficiency with phlegm:

If you have palpitations, diarrhea, insomnia, bloating, gas, indigestion, and you tend to have a lot of phlegm in your throat or post nasal drip or you tend to retain water, with a foggy head especially in humid weather: add Fu Ling (Poria) 20g, Chi Xia Dou and Orange peel10g enhance your digestion and improve your water metabolism. You will sleep better with a healthier heart. You can also drink Barley tea, or you can add Barley30g, daikon30g or wheat germ (30g) into your soup.

5. Liver Blood deficiency:

If you have palpitation with irritability, dry eyes, depression, blurred vision: add Suan Zao Ren 20g (sour Jujube seed) into your soup or porridge.

Acupuncture and acupressure points for irregular heartbeats:

1. Heart and Liver fire with symptoms of irritability, over thinking, feeling warm in the palms and bottoms of the feet:

HT8: On the palm, between the 4th and 5th metacarpal bones. When a fist is made, the point is where the tip of the little finger touches.

KI2: On the medial aspect of the foot, below the tuberosity of the navicular bone, at the junction of the red and white skin.

SI15: 2 cun lateral to the lower border of the spinous process of cervical vertebra seven.

2. Heart and Kidney Yin and blood deficiency: pale complexion, fatigue, dry mouth, thirsty all the time, night sweats or hot flushes, chronic lower back pain, scanty period, dry skin and weak tendons and muscles. Tongue: red, few or peeled coating. Pulse: thin, weak or fast.

Ht6: On the ventral side of the forearm, the point is on the radial side of the tendon m. flexor carpi ulnaris, .5 cun above the transverse crease of the wrist.

CV7: On the anterior median line of the lower abdomen, 1.0 cun below the umbilicus.

CV15: On the anterior median line of the upper abdomen, 1.0 cun below the xiphisternal synchondroses.

3. Qi and Blood stagnation: palpitation with chest tightness and pain, tend to sigh a lot, purple lips and nails, varicose veins, tongue: purple with purple dots, sublingual vein is enlarged and purple, pulse: hesitate, difficulty coming and leaving.

Ht5: On the ventral side of the forearm, the point is on the radial side of the tendon m. flexor carpi ulnaris, 1.0 cun above the transverse crease of the wrist.

Liver 7: on the middle of the medial aspect of the tibia, 7 cun above the tip of the medial malleolus.

PC1: On the chest, in the 4th intercostal space, 1 cun lateral to the nipple.

4. Qi and blood deficiency: difficulty breathing upon exertion, tired all the time, pale complexion, indigestion, tongue: pale with thin white coating, pulse: thin and weak.

SP3: in the depression posterior and inferior to the proximal metatarsodigital joint of the big toe, at the junction of the red and white skin.

CV6: 1.5 cun below belly button, on the front midline of abdomen.

5. Heart Yang and Kidney Yang deficiency: palpitation, fatigue, pale complexion, always feel cold, lower back pain gets better with warm weather, tongue: pale, thin white coating, Pulse: thin and weak.

 GV4: on the posterior median line, in the depression below the spinous process of the 2nd lumbar vertebra.

UB15: On the back, 1.5 cun lateral to the lower border of the spinous process of the 5th thoracic vertebra.

Gao Huang: On the back, 3.0 cun lateral to the lower border of the spinous process of the 4th thoracic vertebra.

Jiu Wei (CV15) On the anterior median line of the upper abdomen, 1.0 cun below the xiphisternal synchondroses (the tip of the sternum).

CV16 (Jiu Que): 6 cun above the belly button, on the midline of the upper abdomen.

KI12: 4 cun bellow bellybutton, 0.5 cun lateral to the front midline.

References

Albanes, D., Weinstein, S.J., Wright, M.E., et al. Serum insulin, glucose, indices of insulin resistance, and risk of prostate cancer. *J. Natl. Cancer Inst.* 2009. 101:1272-1279.

Anastasi, J.K., McMahon, D.J., and Kim, G.H. Symptom management for irritable bowel syndrome: a pilot randomized controlled trial of acupuncture/moxibustion. *Gastroenterol. Nurs.* 2009. 32:243-255.

Bo., C., Zhang, X.S., Huang, H., et al. A study on differences of curative effects of acupuncture and nCPAP for treatment of OSAHS. *Zhongguo Zhen Jiu.* 2008. 28:79-83.

Cabýoglu, M.T., Ergene, N., and Tan, U. The treatment of obesity by acupuncture. *Int. J. Neurosci.* 2006. 116:165-175.

Clementsen, P., Norn, S., Kristensen, K.S., et al. Influenza A virus enhances basophil histamine release and the enhancement is abolished by carbohydrates. *Allergy.* 1990. 45:471-476.

Csoka, A., Bahrick, A., and Mehtonen, O.P. Persistent Sexual Dysfunction after Discontinuation of Selective Serotonin Reuptake Inhibitor. *J. Sex. Med.* 2008. 5: 227-233.

Dean, C.M. *Hormone balance: A Woman's Guide to Restoring Health and Vitality.* 2005. Adams Media Corporation.

Farnsworth, W.E. Roles of estrogen and SHBG in prostate physiology. *Prostate.* 1996. 28:17-23.

Freire, A.O., Sugai, G.C.M., Chrispin, F.S., et al. Treatment of moderate obstructive sleep apnea syndrome with acupuncture: a randomised, placebo-controlled pilot trial. *Sleep Med.* 2007. 8: 43-50.

Gawande, A. Complications: A Surgeon's Notes on an Imperfect Science 2003. Hernry Holt and Company N. Y.

Hecht, K., Vogt, W.F., Wachtel, E., et al. Relationship between insomnia and arterial hypotension. *Pneumologie.* 1991. 45 Suppl 1:196-199.

Jia, C.S., Ma., X.S., Shi, J., et al. Electroacupuncture at Qiuxu (GB 40) for Treatment of Migraine—A Clinical Multicentral Random Controlled Study. *J. Tradit. Chin. Med.* 2009. 29: 43-49.

Jin. P.T. Changes in heart rate, noradrenaline, cortisol and mood during Tai Chi. *J. Psychosom. Res.* 1989. 33:197-206

Jurysta, F., Lanquart, J-P., Van de Borne, P., et al. The link between cardiac autonomic activity and sleep delta power is altered in men with sleep apnea-hypopnea syndrome. *Am. J. Physiol. Regul. Integr. Comp. Physiol.* 2006. 291: 1165-1171.

Lee, J.R. and Hanley, J. *What your doctor may not tell you about premenopause, Balance Your Hormones and Your Life from Thirty and Fifty.* 1999. Warner Wellness.

Li, Y., Liang, F.R., Yang, X.G., et al. Acupuncture for Treating Acute Attacks of Migraine: A Randomized Controlled Trial . *Headache.* 2009. 49:805-816.

Ma, J., Li, H.J., Giovannucci, Ed., et al. Prediagnostic body-mass index, plasma C-peptide concentration, and prostate cancer specific mortality in men with prostate cancer: a long-term survival analysis. *Lancet Oncol.* 2008, 9:1039-1047.

Ma, X.-P., Tan, L.-Y., Yang, Y., et al. Effect of electro-acupuncture on substance P, its receptor and corticotropin-releasing hormone in rats with irritable bowel syndrome. *World J. Gastroenterol.* 2009. 15:5211-5217.

Malek, Z.S., Sage, D., Pevet, P., et al. Daily rhythm of tryptophan hydroxylase-2 messenger ribonucleic acid within raphe neurons Is induced by corticoid daily surge and modulated by enhanced locomotor activity. *Endocrinology.* 2007. 148:5165-5172.

Meltzer, L.J., Logan, D.E., and Mindell, J.A. Sleep patterns in female adolescents with chronic musculoskeletal pain. *Behav. Sleep Med.* 2005. 3:193-208.

Moran, L., and Teede, H. Metabolic features of the reproductive phenotypes of polycystic ovary syndrome. *Human Reproduction Update.* 2009. 15:477-488.

Murray, L., Johnston, B., Lane, A., et al. Relationship between body mass and gastro-oesophageal reflux symptoms: The Bristol Helicobacter Project. *Int. J. Epidemiol.* 2003. 32:645-650.

Omura, Y. Meridian-like networks of internal organs, corresponding to traditional Chinese 12 main meridians and their acupuncture points as detected by the "Bi-Digital O-Ring Test imaging method": search for the corresponding internal organ of Western medicine for each meridian--Part I. *Acupunct. Electrother. Res.* 1987.12:53-70.

Omura, Y. Non-invasive circulatory evaluation and electro-acupuncture & TES treatment of diseases difficult to treat in Western medicine. *Acupunct. Electrother. Res.* 1983. 8:177-256.

Peled, N., Abinader, E. G., Pillar, G., Sharif, D. and Lavie, P. Nocturnal ischemic events in patients with obstructive sleep apnea syndrome and ischemic heart disease: Effects of continuous positive air pressure treatment . 1999. *J. Am. Coll. Cardiol.* 1999. 34: 1744–1749.

Phillips, P.S., Haas, R.H., Bannykh, S., et al. Statin-associated myopathy with normal creatine kinase levels. *Ann. Intern. Med.* 2002. 137:581-585.

Plank, S. and Goodard, J., The Effectiveness of Acupuncture for Chronic Daily Headache: An Outcomes Study *Mil. Med.* 2009. 174: 1276–1281.

Power, A.E. Slow-wave sleep, acetylcholine, and memory consolidation. *Proc. Natl. Acad. Sci. USA.* 2004. 101:1795-1796.

Richards, D. and Marley, J. Stimulation of auricular acupuncture points in weight loss. *Aust. Fam. Physician.* 1998. 27 Suppl. 2:S73-77.

Rye, D.B., and Walters, A.S. Review of the relationship of restless legs syndrome and periodic limb movements in sleep to hypertension heart disease, and stroke. *Sleep.* 2009. 32:589-597.

Schairer, C., McCarty, C.A., Isaacs, C., et al. Circulating insulin-like growth factor (IGF)-I and IGF binding protein (IGFBP)-3 levels and postmenopausal breast cancer risk in the prostate, lung, colorectal, and ovarian cancer screening trial (PLCO) cohort. *Horm Cancer.* 2010. 1:100-111.

Schneider, A., Weiland, C., Enck, P., et al. Neuroendocrinological effects of acupuncture treatment in patients with irritable bowel syndrome. *Complement. Ther. Med.* 2007. 4:255-263.

Spence, D.W., Kayumov, L., Chen, A., et al. Acupuncture increases nocturnal melatonin secretion and reduces insomnia and anxiety: a preliminary report. *J. Neuropsychiatry Clin. Neurosci.* 2004. 16:19-28.

Sugai, G.C., Freire Ade, O., Tabosa, A., et al. Serotonin involvement in the electroacupuncture- and moxibustion-induced gastric emptying in rats. *Physiol. Behav.* 2004. 82:855-861.

Takahashi, T. Acupuncture for functional gastrointestinal disorders. *J. Gastroenterol.* 2006. 41:408-417.

Untersmayr, E., Poulsen, L.K., Platzer, M.H., et al. The effects of gastric digestion on codfish allergenicity. *J. Allergy Clin. Immunol.* 2005. 115:377-382.

Vgontzas, A.N., Tsigos, C., Bixler, E.O., et al. Chronic insomnia and activity of the stress system: a preliminary study. *J. Psychosom. Res.* 1998. 45:21-31.

Voderholzer, U., Hornyak, M., Thiel, B., et al. Impact of experimentally induced serotonin deficiency by tryptophan depletion on sleep EEG in healthy subjects. *Neuropsychopharmacology.* 1998. 18:112-124.

Walters, A. S., and Rye, D.B. Review of the Relationship of Restless Legs Syndrome and Periodic Limb Movements in Sleep to Hypertension, Heart Disease, and Stroke *Sleep.* 2009. 32: 589–597.

Wei, Q., and Liu, Z. Effects of acupuncture on monoamine neurotransmitters in raphe nuclei in obese rats. *J.Tradit. Chin. Med.* 2003. 23:147-150

Winkelman, J.W., and James, L. Serotonergic antidepressants are associated with REM sleep without atonia. *Sleep.* 2004. 27:317-321.

Zou, D., Chen, W.H., Iwakiri, K., et al. Inhibition of transient lower esophageal sphincter relaxations by electrical acupoint stimulation. *Am. J. Physiol. Gastrointest. Liver Physiol.* 2005. 289:197-201.

Index

Made in USA - Kendallville, IN
15818_9798832944418
01.07.2023 1337